YOU'RE NOT A VANITY PURCHASE

YOU'RE
Not a
VANITY
PURCHASE

*Why You Shouldn't Feel Bad
about Looking Good*

JAMES C. MAROTTA, MD, FACS

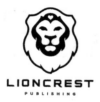

LIONCREST
PUBLISHING

YOU'RE NOT A VANITY PURCHASE

Why You Shouldn't Feel Bad about Looking Good

ISBN   978-1-5445-1822-0 *Hardcover*

   978-1-5445-1821-3 *Paperback*

   978-1-5445-1820-6 *Ebook*

I dedicate this book to my wife, Sharon Marotta. Her never-ending love, support, and encouragement has allowed me to accomplish so many things I could not have otherwise, including this book. Thank you for believing in me more than I do myself sometimes, and thank you for always telling me so. I love you.

Contents

Introduction 9

1. Valerie's Story 15

2. The Guilt and Shame over Plastic Surgery in America:
   For the Vapid, Vain, and Deformed 39

3. Fear: Why Does Plastic Surgery Go Wrong or Too Far? 53

4. The Connection between Looking and Feeling Good 81

5. Changing Your Appearance through Plastic Surgery Is
   Not Giving In to Objectification, Sexism, or Extremism ... 99

6. The Attractiveness Advantage: Why It's Smart to Care
   about How You Look 113

7. The Guilt over Defying Nature: Why Aging "Gracefully"
   Doesn't Always Mean "Naturally" 141

8. Empowering Yourself to Look and Feel the Way You
   Want Safely and Effectively 161

9. Real Patient Stories 181

   Conclusion 187

   Acknowledgments 199

   Appendix: The Most Important Points to Remind
   Yourself of When Doubts Occur 201

   About the Author 211

Introduction

I carve people up for a living. Most of them are women. I make scars, but most of them already have scars before they get to me—scars inflicted deep in their psyche by unwanted attention to a physical flaw. Other times it's because people have stopped paying attention to them altogether. People come to me to change them physically so they can move on mentally.

Here is one of my patient stories: "Since I was a little girl, I have been self-conscious of my nose. This caused extreme stress and contributed to low self-esteem. [I was] made fun of in school; [and my] grades suffered from lack of concentration. [I] made poor choices when starting to date, because I looked for acceptance to compensate for the low self-esteem. [I had a] failed first marriage."

When I asked: "How has surgery changed you? What is your

life like now?" She said: "Surgery has changed my life in such a positive way over the last year. I finally had the confidence to look for another job after twelve years and even accepted an offer. The current job made me a counteroffer to stay with higher pay. I began volunteering at a hospital, visiting the sick. My husband and I remarried in August, which in turn has helped our kids have a stable family. I am able to concentrate on work, family, volunteering, everything!!!

Before the surgery, whether I was driving, giving out communion at church, or holding a training class at work, I was constantly worried about my side view and how everyone saw me. I have now completely cleared my mind of those thoughts. I never worry or think anyone is staring at my nose or how distracting it looks. Those thoughts consumed my life since I was a child, and the freedom and clearer thinking I have now is amazing. It has improved my efficiency at work and increased confidence in my personal life as well."

This is just one patient story about how a physical change can lead to an emotional transformation. Changing someone's appearance can literally change their entire life. I have seen this transformation play out for countless patients who've chosen to undergo plastic surgery or non-surgical enhancement. How many others are out there struggling with their decision to have a procedure? Are you perhaps one of them?

One of the main reasons why people struggle with their

decision to have cosmetic surgery is guilt or shame. How do I know? Because I am a dual-board-certified facial plastic surgeon who listens to people share their struggles every day.

I earned my undergraduate degree at Columbia University. I graduated from medical school with a distinction in research in neuroscience at Stony Brook University. I completed my Head and Neck Surgery residency training at Yale, followed by specialized fellowship training in Facial Plastic Surgery. I have always had a passion for neuroscience and psychology, and the initial reason I went to medical school was to become a psychiatrist. As a facial plastic surgeon, sometimes my job is just that!

I have been in practice for close to fifteen years listening to patients ask: "Am I crazy, doctor? How can I do this to myself? Am I vain? Why do I care so much?" The underlying theme in all of these questions is guilt, and that guilt is pervasive and insidious. It may be accompanied by a good dose of shame, even from a close friend or family member. My answer to these questions usually reassures them: "As long as you're doing this for you, you're not vain," or "There are plenty of other people who feel the same way." While these words of comfort are typically sufficient for patients, they have never truly satisfied me. The unrealized psychiatrist in me wanted to find real answers to their questions, and the curiosity led me to think further: "*Are* they, in fact, being vain? Could they be crazy? Why *do* they care so much?"

This book is the culmination of my experience and research, written to help my patients and any patient out there struggling with guilt or shame over plastic surgery. Perhaps you or someone you know has asked, "Am I being vain?" In this book, I'll answer that question once and for all. I'll also provide better answers, information, and comfort to those wrestling with their decision to have "work done."

This book explores the motivation and drive behind wanting to look good. It examines why the choice to have plastic surgery is often accompanied by much guilt, shame, and fear in the first place. Additionally, it explains why the drive to look one's best is so strong in people of all ages, backgrounds, and persuasions. We will explore the biological, sociological, and psychological reasons people pursue plastic surgery and cosmetic enhancement. As you will discover, people's reasons go way beyond vanity and are much more than "skin deep." We will learn of the power of plastic surgery and aesthetic medicine to transform lives from the outside in. We will discuss why it is not only completely normal to care about the way you look, but downright smart, empowering, and perhaps a healthier way to approach life than you may have previously thought. Finally, we will discuss safe approaches to pursuing cosmetic enhancement and the reality behind plastic surgery "nightmares."

This book is not a comprehensive guide to plastic surgical procedures. Some procedures are mentioned, but if you're looking to find out more about a particular procedure, a web search would better serve your purposes. This book is also not about me or my practice. While I can't help but discuss my personal experience, my background, and even some of the stories of my patients, I did not write this book to sell you on me. Many books written by facial plastic or plastic surgeons are a series of "before" and "after" pictures explaining their surgical philosophy and showcasing their results. This book was not written for that purpose, either.

Most importantly, this book is not intended to sell you on plastic surgery. If you have decided it is not right for you or you would never consider a procedure, I am not here to convince you otherwise. Choosing plastic surgery or non-surgical procedures to change your appearance is a very personal decision. If you object to plastic surgery on the basis of your own morals, beliefs, or ethical grounds, for heaven's sake, put this book down. This book is not an attempt to convert you, although it may. Again, it is written for those struggling with their interest or decision to have plastic surgery. It is for those who are suffering, or feel alone or unsupported in their thinking. I hope this book provides a better answer to all those patients who have asked me over the years: "Am I vain? Why do I do this to myself?" It is a hug, a pat on the back, and support for those people, and hopefully will alleviate any guilt. You should not have to feel bad about wanting to look good. Read on to find out why.

Valerie's Story

*Fear and Judgment: The Story of
a Plastic Surgery Patient*

VALERIE'S STORY

I'd like you to meet Valerie. She's done everything right in life. She worked hard in school, went to the right college, raised a family in a suburb with a good school district, and managed a career to boot. She likes to exercise, as well, and while she prefers yoga, she had spent most of her life on the treadmill. The treadmill she was on was her hectic life: kids off to school, work, laundry, dishes, rinse and repeat. Her kids are off to college now, and the treadmill has at least slowed down enough for her to catch her breath. When she finds time to breathe, though, the breath seems shallower than it should be—not deep, and unfulfilled. The days are a little easier but a lot emptier. The house is quiet.

Valerie is fifty-five now. She turns to her work, and that fills her days. When the alarm goes off, she saunters out of bed and looks in the mirror. She thinks, "Who is that?" She was the high-school homecoming queen and former belle of the ball, but now men barely look at her, including her husband. Over the years, their marriage had grown distant, less affectionate, and less intimate except for special occasions which usually involved drinking. It was hardly the kind of intimacy and affection she craved. She doesn't know how they ended up this way. She doesn't know how it started, whose fault it is, or if it's even anyone's fault. She used to be the kind of girl that turned heads. Now, when she walks in a room, nothing happens, but she occasionally gets hit on by the 85-year-old supermarket patron. That makes her feel good...Not!

Valerie is not a superficial bitch. She knows it's not all about how she looks. She's a smart, accomplished, professional woman. She's well regarded at her investment banking firm, but even there she feels passed over at times. The firm's partners are mostly men, but she's worked and clawed her way up the ladder. It seems like they treat her as one of the guys at this point. Which, she guesses, is a good thing? If she has to hear one more [bleeping] time that she looks tired or is asked if she has gotten enough sleep, she might lose it. The senior partner's face looks like a quilt patchwork with all the blotches and wrinkles he has, but no one asks him that [bleeping] question!

She'll admit the past ten years have not been kind to her or her face. She feels she's aged two decades. Taking care of her aging parents—her mom with Alzheimer's and her father who was in and out of the hospital—had not been easy. The stress took its toll. Both parents passed away within four months.

Valerie's spent her whole life taking care of other people: her kids, her husband, her parents. She's taken care of herself, too. Valerie has got her shit together. She's no wilting lily. She hits the gym, eats right, exercises, and brings home the Benjamins, even more than her husband. She just doesn't know who that person in the mirror is anymore. Her part-ners are right; she does look tired, worn, and, well, old. She's not starting to look like her mom, but for [bleep's] sake, even worse, a little more like her Dad. The bags under her eyes and the "Deputy Dog" look around her mouth and jaw really need to go. She's heard about this plastic surgeon in her area whom a lot of her friends go to. It's worked for them. But she thinks, "Me? Plastic surgery!?" She never thought she'd be there in a million years.

FEAR AND JUDGMENT

Does Valerie's tale sound familiar? Even vaguely? It may not be you; you may not be anything like Valerie. You may be twenty-seven, fifty-seven, or seventy-seven, but some elements of your story are like hers. Chances are if you are reading this book, you're a woman; 90 percent of my patients are. Although if you're not, please don't put the book down or be insulted. You'll find what I am about to say applies to all ages, sexes, proclivities, and orientations. You think you want to make a change through plastic surgery. In fact, it's gotten to the point that you know you have to, but you don't know where to turn to get information about the fear, doubt, guilt, or shame you're experiencing.

You may fear being judged for thinking about plastic surgery. You may judge yourself. Your inner voice might say: "I am being vain and weak. After all, vanity is one of the seven deadly sins, is it not? I am committing a sin by thinking this way. I should be more self-reliant and self-confident. A stronger person would be happier in their own skin. A stronger person would use their inner beauty to overcome their external flaws." You may be wrestling with this thinking internally, and you will also find plenty of people in your closest circles who echo this sentiment. They may not be as direct, but comments like "I like you just the way you are" and "Why can't you just be happy with yourself?" are subtle or not-so-subtle hints that the person thinks you are vain and need to get a grip.

Financial judgment is another theme I see commonly. With cosmetic procedures, people worry they are being frivolous with their money. Let's face it, if you go to someone with excellent credentials, experience, and artistry, it's not cheap. Some people feel they can't justify spending so much money on a "vanity" purchase. The financial guilt with regard to cosmetic procedures seems to apply to people at all levels of income or wealth. Whether I am dealing with a retired postal worker spending part of her life savings or a multimillionaire for whom the expense is a mere drop in the bucket, there is the same financial remorse. If they're having trouble justifying the expense to themselves, the fear of accusations from their partners, spouses, family, and friends can be overwhelming. They actually hear or anticipate hearing things like, "You want to spend how much on a facelift?" Somehow, spending on other things (like a ridiculously priced handbag or pair of shoes) doesn't seem to spark the same contempt or indignation from people as spending money to alter appearance.

You may be overwhelmed by fear or anxiety regarding the procedure and its potential outcome. The very core of any fear is to avoid danger, and that is the reason you are fearful. Plastic surgery procedures, even the non-invasive kind, do have risks. But in the hands of a qualified practitioner, is plastic surgery dangerous? Not really. The unknown conjures all kinds of scenarios in our minds, but fears are usually disproportionate to the actual risk. "What if I have a complication? What if I go blind, I lose part of my face, my nose falls off (à la Michael Jackson), or I die under anesthesia?" These are the kinds of questions that may be swirling around in your head, and they're questions I commonly hear from my patients.

While having a disastrous medical complication is one thing, you may be equally frightened about the potential results. "What if I come out looking weird or unnatural? What is the deal with these celebrities who have so much money, access to the best plastic surgeons, and yet come out looking like unrecognizable freaks? What about Kenny Rogers, Joan Rivers, Mickey Rourke, Donatella Versace, or (insert celebrity name here)?"

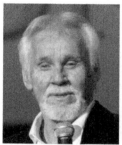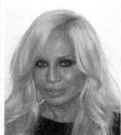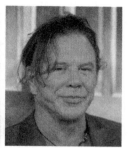

Left: Alamy photographer: Zuma. Center: Alamy photographer: dpa. Right: Alamy photographer: unknown

Even if you aren't worried about this kind of extreme, you may just be concerned that you may not like the way things turn out. This may be the most insidious fear you have as a plastic surgery patient. The reality is, at some point you have to just put your faith and trust in your surgeon's hands, which is, well, *scary*.

VALERIE'S CHOICE

Now back to Valerie's story. Valerie does what any reasonable woman would do in her shoes; she turns to Google. She Googles a local doctor. He has mostly great reviews. There are a few angry ones, too, but they sound like crazies. She looks at his before-and-after gallery on the website. "Hmmm…I kind of look like her. Wow, she looks fabulous. Very natural, but ten to fifteen years younger. That's what I want." Valerie gets up the courage to call, but she hangs up because she realizes she's in her office at work. She's behind her closed door in her corner office, but she's still worried. What if her executive assistant overhears? Oh God, maybe they go through the phone calls and internet searches. Will someone see where she called or see what she Googled? She decides to call later from her car on her cell phone during the commute home.

During her drive, she gets up the courage to call again. With her heart pounding and her breath quickened, she is greeted by a very friendly, confident voice on the other side of the phone. She gets the sense this person has probably talked another version of herself off the ledge before. She is unsure of exactly what procedure she needs or wants, or exactly what she wants to change. The woman guides her seamlessly through a series of questions and helps her book her consult date. She did it! She took the first step. The hardest part of that whole process was making the phone call in the first place.

Sure, she had a bunch of medical jargon swirling through her head from her Google search: Deep Plane Facelift, Juvederm, and Fractional Laser Resurfacing. She thought she would impress her phone mate with her newfound knowledge, but in reality, she had no clue what those things really meant. She started the phone call that way, but the patient-care coordinator could tell she was bluffing to impress. The coordinator assured her that she would receive the knowledge she needed during the consultation, and that was enough.

Valerie goes home after a long day, uncorks a nice red, and toasts to her bravery. "Tomorrow's a new day," she thinks, and drifts off into a deep slumber.

A week later, Valerie finds herself at dinner with her husband, Michael. She can't believe her consultation with the doctor is coming next week. She doesn't quite know how to broach the subject or if she should even tell him. Their communication hasn't been the greatest lately, nor has Michael been sympathetic to what she is going through. Every time she's mentioned her discontent over her appearance, he's brushed her off. "You look fine… I don't know what you're talking about." As if he would know—he hasn't looked at her for at least five years. But she's never had the kind of marriage where she's kept secrets. She doesn't need his permission to do anything, but she doesn't like hiding things either, no matter how he might react.

"So, Michael," she begins. "You know I haven't been happy with the way I am aging. I made an appointment to see a doctor about plastic surgery."

"What? Have you lost your mind? We have two kids in college. Do you know what that costs? Are you really that self-absorbed? A woman of your age and achievements. Why the hell do you care!? I don't care what you look like." Valerie thinks, "That's for sure."

Michael starts again, "Why would you do something like this by choice? What if something happens? You know people die doing that stuff. And what if you come out looking like a freak? I have seen a few women in Manhattan with that stuff, and let me tell you! Think about those celebrities you've seen that have had it done."

Valerie's had it. She feels crushed. and she's ready to give up on the whole idea. "I'll just continue to hate the way I look," she thinks. Later, she turns to her sister, who surely would understand. But her sister is five years younger. Surprisingly, she runs into the same stonewall and barrage of frantic questions: "Why would you even think of something like this? I know your friends are doing this stuff, but if they jumped off a bridge, would you do it too? I don't know, Sis, I'm just worried about you. I don't think plastic surgery is a good idea. Why don't you try the natural way?"

Frustrated and feeling alone, with no support from her family, she calls her best friend whose acquaintance, Donna, had something done. She wants to arrange a call, but the woman offers to meet her in person. They meet for lunch and talk about Valerie's situation. Donna is so kind, so open. Donna tells her, "I ran into the same thing; I was actually berated by my sister. Easy for her to say—she is ten years younger! My husband wasn't exactly supportive either, but I had it a little easier with him. He just said, 'Whatever you want to do, babe.' Look, I can tell you on the other side of this thing, my only regret is that I didn't do it sooner. It has literally changed my life." She tells Valerie exactly what she had done: a facelift, upper and lower eyelids, and fat injections. She shows her the scars to prove it, although Valerie has a hard time seeing anything resembling a scar. She thought they would be a lot worse. Donna even offers to come to the consultation with Valerie.

THE NEXT STEP

Valerie decides to take Donna up on her offer. She keeps her appointment with the doctor. She goes to the office and immediately feels she is in the right place. Everyone she meets at the office is friendly and engaging. They are not "salesy," but rather they have a "we are here to help you" attitude. She first meets with the patient-care coordinator, Sandra, who explains that her job is to guide Valerie through the process from start to finish. Sandra asks Valerie:

"So why are you here? What bothers you when you look in the mirror?" She lists the credentials of the doctor and the practice, and Valerie is blown away by the experience this guy has. She looks at before-and-after pictures and loves what she sees. Everyone looks better, ten to fifteen years younger, but in a natural way. She would have no clue that they had "plastic surgery" because there is nothing plastic about these faces.

She meets the doctor, and he is very pleasant and kind. She feels a little nervous, but he puts her at ease. He asks her if she brought the pictures of herself in which she last liked the way she looked, as he requested. The doctor reviews the pictures and describes the changes he sees in her appearance. He does a physical exam and then makes his recommendations, presenting multiple treatment options to address her concerns. They talk about what she should expect for downtime and recovery for each of the different options. Valerie has plenty of time she can take off from work as she hasn't used many vacation days since the kids have left the house. The doctor then shows her a series of before-and-after results with faces similar to hers. He steps out of the room to allow Valerie to discuss her options with the patient-care coordinator, including scheduling and pricing.

Valerie ultimately decides to have full facial rejuvenation, an upper and lower blepharoplasty (eyelid lift), brow lift, facelift, fat injections, and laser skin resurfacing: "the works." She figures she might as well do it once and do it right. She doesn't want to discuss it with Michael or her sister. She doesn't care, because she is doing this for herself. And having Donna there for moral support gives her the courage to go through with it. She picks the date and calls her administrative assistant to schedule the time off work.

A few days later, she's at home, and she decides she has to tell Michael. "Whether you support me or not, I am doing this," Valerie says. Michael surprises her. Although he still thinks she is making a mistake, he agrees to support her going forward. He drives her to her preoperative appointment and hears what she is actually having done. At that visit, a nurse goes over medications, postoperative care, and more of what to expect. Michael is more than a little freaked out because he heard none of this the first go-around. The doctor comes in and reviews the potential complications, or, as Michael anxiously hears it, "all the things that could go wrong." The doctor reassures them that the risks are small, and complications are relatively rare, but there are still risks. Michael thinks of using this as ammunition against having the procedures, but then decides to stay supportive and committed to help Valerie through. He can be a good nurse for a couple of days. Besides, he could use some time off of work too.

THE BIG DAY

The day of the surgery, the couple are both basket cases: Valerie has nervous excitement, while Michael is just plain nervous. They arrive at the doctor's office early. Michael can't believe they have operating rooms at the office and they don't have to go to the hospital. They are greeted by the nurse they met at the preoperative appointment, a friendly, familiar face. They are taken into an exam room. The nurse takes Valerie's vital signs, asks her some questions, and then asks her to change into a gown. The anesthesiologist, who called them the night before, comes in and introduces himself. He seems very confident and competent. He goes over the kind of anesthesia Valerie is going to have and then talks about the risks. Michael thinks, "Why do these guys talk about this stuff so much if it is 'so unlikely' to happen?'"

The surgeon comes in and marks up Valerie's face like a road map. He puts her hair in little pigtails, and she looks ridiculous. Michael threatens a picture for social media, and Valerie threatens much worse retaliation if he does. The laughing helps calm their nerves. The doctor leaves, and the nurse returns. Michael holds Valerie's hand for the first time in a while, a very long while. As she is ready to be taken back to surgery, Michael hugs Valerie and kisses her goodbye. Valerie wonders what has gotten into him. Why the sudden change? But she is grateful she didn't have to go through this without him.

Michael spends the next five hours pacing the local Starbucks and frantically banging out emails for work. It keeps him busy but not distracted. All he can think about is Valerie. Is she okay? What is taking so long? Finally, he receives a phone call from the doctor, who tells him everything went great, and Valerie is in the recovery room. He quickly grabs his keys and heads back to the office, which is only fifteen minutes away. He waits another half hour, and the nurse brings him back to the recovery area to see Valerie.

Michael sees her and almost collapses. The nurse told him about the bandages, the swelling, and the bruising, but what he saw was his worst fear. Valerie doesn't even look like his wife. She looks like some alien or avatar, and her wide, puffed-out face surrounded by so much gauze makes her head look like a living Q-tip. Oh God, there are "drains" taped to the side of her head. Pipes with blood. The nurses told him about all of this stuff, but seeing it is nearly overwhelming. The nurse assures him this is all normal.

Valerie is gorked out and having a grand old time. She sounds like the Valerie that had one too many. She is a little too loose-lipped and starts asking Michael, "Now that I look beautiful, would you like to try me out again?" "Yeah, right," he thinks. He knew she shouldn't have added on that laser resurfacing at the last moment. Maybe that's why she is so swollen? The nurses assure him again that this is all normal, and they review the medications with an easy-to-use, color-coded system. They review drain care…gulp. He doesn't want to do any of this stuff and is not quite sure he has the stomach for it. It seems the nurse almost reads the look of concern in his eyes and encourages him: "Every little thing we talked about is spelled out for you right here on these few sheets. You got this. If you have any questions, we are always here to help. Just give us a call." The nurse helps him get Valerie into the car, as she is certainly in no condition to do so herself.

On the drive home, he glances over at her, and all of his fears resurface. Michael thinks, "I had to be out of my mind to let her go through with this. What was I thinking? Hell, what was *she* thinking? I knew she would come out looking like a totally different person." Fortunately, Michael is smart enough to maintain his composure for Valerie's sake and keeps his mouth shut. At home, his job as nurse begins, and he gets her into bed. He has a restless night of sleep while Valerie snores in a drugged-up slumber.

AFTERWARD

They awake the next morning. Well, Michael never really actually slept. They hightail it to the doctor's office for an appointment at 10 a.m., and they are greeted by the recovery-room nurse from the day before. She is a welcome, familiar face. The nurse starts taking off the bandages and reviewing the postoperative care. Surprisingly Michael feels completely confident. It's really not that hard, and now's he's heard it for the third time. "Apply peroxide and antibiotic ointment to the suture lines twice a day...blah, blah, blah." Ugh...the suture lines. As the nurse unwraps the bandages, he realizes Valerie actually looks worse today, if that is even possible. Like some puffy Pillsbury Doughboy. He wonders if that is the look she was going for, and he chuckles to himself. As if she were reading his mind, the nurse looks at him, smiles, and says, "This is all completely normal."

The doctor enters the room. He does a quick physical exam, then confidently states that everything is looking great. Michael thinks to himself: "This is what you call 'looking great'?" Valerie is comfortable except for the fact that she is having a little trouble opening her swollen eyes to see anything. She is surprised to hear the doctor say the swelling could be worse tomorrow. She wonders, "How can I possibly be any more swollen than this?" The doctor gives her a few shots of lidocaine, a numbing anesthetic, and painlessly removes the drains. He reviews her post-operative care to make sure they are clear on everything. Valerie is just so happy the surgery is over and that she actually went through with it. She hopes it turns out as she imagined, but she won't let her mind go there right now. She is just looking forward to getting home and sleeping some more. The doctor tells her good nutrition, sleep, and relaxation are the keys to a rapid recovery. She is totally onboard with that program, but a chocolate milkshake can't hurt in the mix. They go home, and Valerie sleeps for the rest of the day.

Valerie doesn't have another follow-up appointment until "postop day three." She is even learning the doctor lingo. "Postop day zero" is the day of the operation, and then each successive day is counted from there. The doctor was right, the next day the swelling is even worse. It looks as if her cheeks could be popped like a balloon. By the second day, the swelling in her eyelids has come down at least enough for her to see. After a few more days, the swelling gets much better. She shows up for her appointment and has her eyelid sutures taken out. While it didn't really hurt, it wasn't exactly fun either. The doctor was right; she really doesn't feel much pain. Her face has this weird kind of numbness, and her remaining face/brow lift sutures are starting to itch. As the days go by, she sees small, encouraging signs of improvement. The swelling and the bruising are going down little by little. Although Valerie is starting to recognize her own face, she is not exactly thrilled with what she sees. But she trusts the doctor and the nurses, who repeatedly assure her that she is still pretty swollen.

TWO WEEKS LATER

Now that two weeks have passed, Valerie is wondering why she did this. While she is looking better, even more like herself, when she looks in the mirror, all she can see is the purple still left, the lump by her right cheek, the scars around her ears, and the scars on her eyelids. "Christ...what was I thinking?" she sobs gently to herself in her bathroom. Michael comes in, and she tries to catch herself and hold it back, but she can't. "What the hell is wrong with you?" he snaps. Michael has had it. It's been a long two weeks for him, too. He was happy when his nursing duties were over, and was able to escape back to work on day five. Valerie replies: "I don't know if I did the right thing. Look at me. I mean, my neck and jaw are beautiful, but I still look like I have these big wide cheeks, and my eyes are still puffy." Michael erupts. "You know, I've held it in for two weeks. I went with you to all your appointments, gave you your medicines, and got you out of bed during those first two days. But I can't take it anymore. I told you not to do this. Don't like the way you look? That's your f*cking fault." Michael leaves. A torrent of guilt and regret washes over Valerie, and she sobs uncontrollably. She feels utterly alone.

After a good twenty-minute cry, Valerie looks in the mirror. "Oh God, I didn't think it was possible, but now I look even more puffy." She puts on her sweats, darns her big sunglasses and hoodie, and heads out for her two-week follow-up appointment. She is going to see the doctor, but the medical assistant comes in first. Valerie frenetically unleashes her torrent of questions in rapid-fire succession: "Am I still supposed to be bruised at this point? Am I still swollen? Why are the scars so red and itchy? Why do my eyes still look glassy? Is this the way I am going to look?" The medical assistant does her best to calm Valerie and brings in the doctor.

Before she can start, the doctor, as if knowing what is coming, says, "I understand you have a bunch of questions and concerns. Let's talk about them." Valerie unloads, "What about...?" Normal. "And...?" Normal. "And also...?" Normal. The doctor assures her that she is progressing quite nicely and reminds her that although the major part of recovery is in the first few days, significant healing and changes would still take place over the next month. Then he says, "Valerie, it is not uncommon for people to feel downright depressed at the two-week mark from surgery and even have some major regrets." Valerie thinks, "Wait, did he bug my bathroom?" He reminds her of something that was tucked away in her preoperative packet of information. A single-page sheet that says, "Two weeks after surgery, you may feel down, depressed, and regret that you did this." The doctor gives her another sheet and reviews that there is a physiologic reason as to why she may feel down at this point: her fight-or-flight hormones have been depleted from the two weeks of healing, anxiety, and less-than-perfect sleep. Valerie gets the sense he's been here before with thousands of people and had this same conversation with them. She leaves the office feeling better and a bit more confident. Or, at least, not completely alone.

Michael is back home again. He is distant and cold when she walks in. She approaches him and tells him she feels better. She is going to be patient and explains her experience at the doctor's office. Michael turns and apologizes. He says part of him is just worried that she won't be happy after all this. He says he sees a lot of good things from the surgery, but agrees there is still some stuff that looks, well, weird.

Valerie plans to return to work on Monday, which is postop day sixteen. She knows she is still swollen, but the makeup they showed her at the office really helps. She practices on Sunday, concealing the evidence. When she is done with her makeup, she stares long and hard. "Holy crap," she thinks, "I actually look pretty good." She sees her eyes for the first time since the surgery. The eyeshadow actually goes on her upper eyelids and doesn't smear or run. While she is using a little concealer for her lower eyelids to cover the last remnants of bruising, it pales in comparison to the amount she used to cake on to cover her bags and dark circles. Her jawline and neck look tight and youthful. She hates to even think of the "jowls" she had two weeks ago. What a gross expression. Well, anyway, her jowls are gone. The doctor told her that her face is a little swollen even now from the fat injections, so she knows her cheeks are a little bigger than they're going to be in the end. Michael sees her for the first time with some makeup on. "Wow. I have to admit, babe, you look incredible. You look like you did fifteen years ago." Valerie thinks, "Babe? He hasn't called me anything, let alone 'Babe,' in months." She catches Michael staring, lost in thought for a moment. She hardly feels attractive right now, but Michael lingers and looks at her again before leaving the room. Valerie feels like this is the first time he's really seen her in years.

AMAZING RESULTS

Valerie goes to work the next day. She is a nervous wreck and knows people are going to notice. She just hopes people don't stare too long or make her feel uncomfortable. She didn't really advertise what she was doing. "It's no one else's business," she thought. She goes to her morning meeting with the partners. She is greeted warmly by each. "I guess absence makes the heart grow fonder at work, too," she thinks. She hears, "Wow, you look great! Vacation really agreed with you. Did you do something to your hair?" (She did, by the way, to throw some interference). "Did you lose weight?" each partner and administrator she runs into asks. The odd thing is they seem really sincere. Could they really have no clue what she did? Valerie works the full day, and it actually feels good to be back to work. The strange thing is, she not only looks different, but *feels* different at work. She feels more centered, more engaging. People seem to react to her differently, as well. It was way easier to be heard at the meeting this morning. She felt on her game, and whatever she said seemed to be received differently than it was three weeks ago.

Months go by and Valerie goes to the doctor for her six-month postoperative visit. Everything has changed on the outside as well as the inside. The scars have faded to nothing over the past few months. Even without makeup on, the scars are no longer visible. The swelling and even the "extra" fat the doc put in her cheeks have gone down considerably. The lumps and bumps and the numbness she felt over the past couple of months are pretty much gone. She feels completely healed, although the doctor said things will continue to improve over the course of a year. The doctor does an examination and tells her the healing is proceeding nicely. In fact, Valerie looks so good, he thought she might enjoy seeing her before-and-after pictures. Valerie nearly falls off the chair. She cannot believe what she looked like before. She can't believe she walked around like that for so long. She can't believe she felt so badly about herself for so many years.

In the months since her surgery, Valerie feels like a different person. She's more confident, more comfortable in her own skin, and more like her old self. In fact, when she looks at pictures of herself from fifteen years ago, she pretty much looks exactly like *that*—her old self. Her relationship with Michael is completely different. Because she feels more comfortable, he became more interested. First, it was the longer glances, then the staring. Then the more intimate moments which multiplied into something else... an entirely different relationship. They've become husband and wife again instead of just housemates. Her career has taken off, too. She's brought in more big clients to the firm in the past six months than she did over the past two years. People seem to react to her differently. It's just easier to close deals now. She has a newfound passion for her work.

As she stares at the before-and-after pictures, the tears well up in her eyes. She remembers the flood of emotions she went through to even get to the procedure table. The fear, the doubt, the guilt—oh, the guilt. And it was made even worse by the people she loved the most in her life, Michael and her sister.

Valerie's life and appearance were transformed through her cosmetic procedures. The same is true for many other women who take the leap of faith and make the changes they long for. The question is, why does the choice have to be so difficult? Why do people, such as Valerie, face fear, shame, guilt, and even remorse about cosmetic procedures? What is it about making a change to one's appearance that invites such trepidation, doubt, and even outright scorn by the people around you? We'll explore the origins of the guilt and fear surrounding plastic surgery in the next few chapters.

2

The Guilt and Shame over Plastic Surgery in America: For the Vapid, Vain, and Deformed

So why do Valerie and millions of people like her have such mental anguish about wanting to improve their appearance? Why such guilt and shame? When you think about plastic surgery or non-surgical procedures, what do you think about? Are the images and thoughts that occur to you positive or negative?

While the thoughts and opinions that individuals hold on the subject are as widely varied as any, the typical American view on plastic surgery is overwhelmingly negative. The general consensus is that plastic surgery is scary and macabre. Plastic surgery is for people who are vain and are not happy with the person they are inside. Plastic surgery is for vapid people who are superficial and care about their looks too much. Plastic surgery leads to people looking weird, and if you get it, you are going to look weird too.

I have worked in this field for over fifteen years and have heard these sentiments echoed again and again by more people than I care to count. In fact, some of these thoughts are the very first thing out of people's mouths when they learn what I do. And I imagine people are holding back a bit when they express their opinions to me, a facial plastic surgeon who has made changing people's faces his life's work. I encounter negative opinions about plastic surgery even from the patients who are in my office pursuing cosmetic enhancement. I would imagine those who wouldn't step foot in a plastic surgeon's office have even stronger negative views. Given the generally negative consensus, it is not surprising that people considering cosmetic enhancement might run into a potential chorus of social condemnation and even shaming. In this chapter, we'll explore the origins of the negativity and guilt surrounding plastic surgery.

WHAT DOES "PLASTIC" MEAN TO YOU?

Part of the public-relations problem for Plastic Surgery may be in its very name. People associate the word "plastic" with something manufactured, fake, or phony. Just like the material plastic, anything created with plastic surgery is, by extension, "manufactured," man-made, inferior, or defective. The word has such a negative connotation that "plastic" is often used to refer to people who have had plastic surgery that others view as unnatural or over the top. But the "plastic" in plastic surgery has nothing to do with the material, a fake appearance, or being man-made. "Plastic" comes from the Greek word *plastikos*, meaning "to mold or change." Plastic surgery is quite literally and simply the art of molding or changing the body through surgery.

AMERICAN VALUES AND VIEWS

Beyond the name, what are some of the other reasons why Americans might have guilt or shame over plastic surgery? For one thing, as progressive as the United States can be, conservative, Christian values are still at the core of American culture. The influence of these values makes us, as a culture, a lot more uptight about the human body and conflicted about whether or not we should be allowed to change it. From the very founding of the nation, Protestantism and its offshoots (e.g., Puritanism, Presbyterianism, and Calvinism) became the dominant religions in the United States. Puritans believed in the doctrine of predestination. In this doctrine, God's will, not human behavior, determines whether a person will be saved or damned. Calvinists believed in predetermination, meaning every event in the course of human history was purposefully orchestrated and "predetermined" by God.

In addition, the Protestant religions that dominated American culture were a lot more suspicious of the human body than their European counterparts. They covered it up and concealed it (think Pilgrim). They avoided beautifying and adorning it (think Puritan). They viewed the human form as a vehicle for the devil to lure them into sin. In Christian theology, the body is just a vessel, a mere piece of clothing to be eventually discarded. The soul is our elevated, true self. It is the only really important part of us, and it's what continues to live on in the afterlife. The body and soul are separate entities. Christianity informs us that in all circumstances, our focus and intention should be on the soul and not the body.

How might our "Puritanical" views as Americans color our thinking about altering our bodies with plastic surgery? It makes us a lot more conflicted and guilt-ridden about altering what God gave us. If we were created by a God who is perfect, who are we to go and change that? If we have physical flaws, he or she may have done that with intention. The events of our lives related to those physical flaws may be part of a greater plan (predetermination). Perhaps those physical flaws are meant to present us with challenges in life that we are supposed to overcome. Being teased about a big nose, bat ears, or tires under our eyes may build stronger moral character. Perhaps these social challenges are ways of directing us to a greater good. If you are not capable of overcoming these physical flaws, you are vain; you're not a strong or moral person.

To focus too much on outward physical appearance is human—even worse, the work of the devil (Puritanism). If you are focused on someone's physical beauty, you are being lustful. If you focus on your own beauty, you are being vain. Our Christian values tell us the moral thing to do is to "see" another person's soul and not their outward physical appearance. People should be capable of seeing beyond any physical flaw or external cue if they are good. If they are sinful and prone to the devil's enticements, they make the body more important than it should be.

"It's what's inside that counts." Ever heard that before? It is such a common expression in American vernacular that it's hard to imagine its origins in religion. As Americans, we are more guilt-ridden and uptight about altering our appearance through plastic surgery, and that is partially because of our shared American values. These shared American values stem from our colonial beginnings as a predominantly Puritan society.

REALITY TV: PLASTIC SURGERY IS FOR THE VAPID

Guilt over cosmetic surgery is also prevalent in America because of how plastic surgery is portrayed in the media. Plastic surgery is a favored subject of reality TV. After all, who does this stuff? The Real Housewives and the Kardashians, that is who. How do these shows represent these people? Drama, drama, drama. They are not real people. They are caricatures of real people. Now I do not know any of them personally, nor have I ever watched these shows for more than thirty seconds in flipping the channels, but I would say it's a safe bet that some of the extreme behavior, the hedonism, the vanity, and the self-centered, self-absorbed displays are exaggerated, made for TV, and scripted. I would hope these reality TV stars are a little more centered than the shows paint them to be.

How are these stars viewed by the general public? Certainly not as pillars of normal, moral behavior, but as outlandish, spoiled, self-absorbed, and, well, vain. The entire entertainment value of these shows is for people to sit there and judge, and to make them feel better about themselves. "I may not have as much money as those people, but at least I'm normal. These people are crazy." The regular visits of reality TV stars to plastic surgeons and the cosmetic treatments featured on their shows reinforce that they are the typical plastic surgery patient: vapid, vain, and "over the top." Nothing could be further from the truth.

Some shows portray plastic surgery not only as vanity but downright insanity. Remember the show *Extreme Makeover*? Even the title says to everyone watching that plastic surgery is "extreme." There was also a similar show called *The Swan*. On both of these shows, patients had a massive number of procedures with the goal of creating a radical transformation for the climax or "big reveal." The point of these shows was for the contestant to come out looking completely different, like the ugly duckling who changed into the swan. These misleading portrayals feed into the macabre and creepy notion that plastic surgery radically changes people's identity.

REALITY TV: A FOCUS ON THE SENSATIONAL, THE NEGATIVE ELEMENTS, AND THE DANGER

Another negative plastic surgery stereotype reinforced by reality TV is danger. Reality TV focuses on the sensationalism and the danger in plastic surgery. Rock singer Gene Simmons showcased his facelift on an episode of *Gene Simmons Family Jewels* in 2007. In this episode, he had a complication following his procedure: a hematoma. A hematoma is a blood collection underneath the skin following a facelift. It rarely happens, but is more common in males and in people with high blood pressure. Complications, in general, are very rare following plastic surgery, and a hematoma is easily treatable and doesn't affect the long-term outcome. The episode, of course, focused more on the gore, blood, and drains coming out of Simmons's head than on the long-term result. I guess it was fun for everyone watching to say, "Well, I guess he deserved it for getting plastic surgery."

If you don't believe the notion that plastic surgery on reality TV is portrayed in a mostly negative light, consider the title of today's most popular plastic surgery reality TV show, *Botched*. Who makes it on the show? Patients on the fringes and extremes of plastic surgery with surgical disasters. Those who did something crazy in the first place like inject their own silicone or motor oil into their bodies. Those who traveled abroad and had surgery in a garage. Those who are on their fifth or sixth surgery on the same body part. Those who want to look like a cartoon character or an animal and have intentionally disfigured themselves. Reality TV portrays plastic surgery like a three-ring circus with a never-ending cast of crazy, side-show freakish characters rather than a medical profession that deals with real people and real problems.

The medical profession clearly recognized that reality TV presents a problem for plastic surgery in America. A 2007 article entitled "Plastic Surgery Is Real, Not Reality TV" in the *AMA Journal of Ethics* by Dr. Richard D'Amico stated: "Illustrating real-life plastic surgery experiences as a form of entertainment has trivialized the practice of cosmetic plastic surgery. While reality TV shows increase public awareness about the latest surgery options, they have created a troublesome byproduct—unrealistic and unhealthy expectations in potential patients. It is crucial for patients to understand that plastic surgery is real surgery with real risks. Further, the introduction of entertainment into reality-based plastic surgery programs has tarnished the image of the profession."

So, we've established that as a culture, America's views of plastic surgery and those who pursue it are not usually positive. Despite the progressive nature of our society, we are more culturally conservative when it comes to beautification through alteration. There is more guilt and shame associated with cosmetic surgery in America, which is most likely the result of our origins as a conservative Christian (Puritanical) society. The negative stigma around plastic surgery is further deepened by the media's portrayal of cosmetic surgery on reality TV, the internet, and tabloids. Vain, immoral people prone to drama choose it. Celebrities end up disfigured from it. You will likely end up with a complication, or worse, dead from it.

A DIFFERENT PERSPECTIVE

If you look back at history and at the majority of cultures throughout the world, you will find an entirely different view of plastic surgery and the pursuit of physical beauty. Worlds away from the negative portrayals on reality TV is a view that is guilt-free, life-affirming, and overwhelmingly positive. The ancient Egyptians regarded physical beauty and the pursuit of it as a sign of holiness, not of evil or sin. Everything they used to improve their physical appearance had not only an aesthetic significance but a magical and religious importance. For example, their makeup palettes were in the shape of a fish, which is the symbol of resurrection and new life. These beautification tools were thought to be so important to the soul that they were placed in Ancient Egyptian tombs alongside gold.

The Ancient Greeks also venerated the human body and equated physical beauty with the divine. They believed their gods had human form and were depicted in Greek statues as having the ultimate athletic bodies. These statues filled their marketplaces, meeting places, and temples. In Ancient China, the religions placed a huge emphasis on the relationship between female inner and outer beauty.[1] Outer beauty was thought to represent virtuousness, talent, and other positive characteristics. The various Chinese dynasties throughout history created female beauty ideals, which were pursued by women as a sign of morality.

The idea that focusing on physical beauty is sinful or vain is a complete 180-degree turn from the way improving one's appearance was perceived throughout history. Since the beginning of time, human beings have been engaged in making themselves appear more beautiful. For this reason, plastic surgery may be one of the world's oldest healing arts.[2]

To give some examples, plastic surgery began in Ancient Egypt. The repair of a broken nose was described in a transcription of an Ancient Egyptian medical text on a papyrus dated back to 3000 to 2500 BC. Aulus Cornelius Celsus, a

---

1   https://en.wikipedia.org/wiki/Chinese_ideals_of_female_beauty

2   https://www.verywellhealth.com/the-history-of-plastic-surgery-2710193

first-century Roman, described the first eyelid lift in which excisions of skin were made to relax the eyelids.[3] As far back as 1845, Friedrich Dieffenbach from Germany described the first official "nose job" by the reduction of a "large, hanging nose."

PLASTIC SURGERY AROUND THE WORLD

Plastic surgery and physical enhancement have had a very long history. They were not associated with evil, but with the divine and holy, and have never really had an image problem except in modern America. In many cultures throughout the world, plastic surgery is celebrated and even venerated as life-affirming, empowering, and without negative bias or associations. Plastic surgery in Brazil is truly a cultural phenomenon. In many cities, undergoing cosmetic surgery is a rite of passage. It is a regular topic of conversation among all sectors of the population, and cosmetic surgeons are often regarded as celebrities. In fact, Ivo Pitanguay, the famous plastic surgeon, carried Brazil's torch in the 2016 Olympics.

In Brazil, enhancing sex appeal through plastic surgery is a most common goal. Breast augmentations and the "Brazilian Butt Lift" which augments the buttocks with fat are popular procedures. In the Far East, according to statistics provided by the International Society of Aesthetic Plastic Surgery, South Korea has the most cosmetic surgery per

---

3   https://en.wikipedia.org/wiki/De_Medicina

capita. One in five women in Seoul, Korea, has had plastic surgery. Plastic surgery is a widely accepted and celebrated undertaking. For example, a typical high-school graduation gift for a teenager is the gift of a nose job or double eyelid surgery.[4]

Europeans have an entirely different view of plastic surgery, even in culturally religious or Catholic societies where you might think plastic surgery would be viewed as vain or sinful. In Italy, for example, plastic surgery is quite popular. It is no secret that Italians like to *fare una Bella figura*, which is translated "make a beautiful appearance." The former prime minister Silvio Berlusconi had a facelift and a hair transplant. Could you imagine an American president or candidate admitting to that? In Greece, where nudity is celebrated in Ancient Greek sculpture, it's not surprising that penis enlargements are performed ten times more often than the world average. France has always been at the center of the beauty industry, and Belgium has a higher rate of plastic surgery per capita than the US.

In Northern Africa and the Middle East, some of the most ardently religious societies like Libya, Iran, Egypt, and Saudi Arabia view cosmetic surgery in a positive light, and it is quite popular in these cultures. Muammar Al Gadhafi, the former prime minister of Libya, had several procedures done, including Botox, fillers, and a facelift. Whether a

---

4   https://www.newyorker.com/magazine/2015/03/23/about-face

rhinoplasty in Beirut, breast augmentation in Dubai, or tummy tucks in Turkey, plastic surgery is wildly popular in the Middle East. The highest number of plastic surgeons per capita, even greater than Beverly Hills, can now be found in Dubai.

I quote these world statistics not to give the impression that cosmetic surgery is not popular in the US. The United States, by sheer population size and wealth, still has the most cosmetic procedures done in the world per year. On a per-capita basis, however, the US only ranks sixth in the world. Clearly, the public-relations problem, the bias, and the guilt and shame associated with plastic surgery have some impact on American people feeling free to pursue it. But as you have seen here, the negative attitude that most Americans have toward plastic surgery is an oddity in the world. And even though some of America's contention with plastic surgery and altering one's appearance has a basis in moral or religious objections, there are plenty of fervently religious cultures (e.g., the Middle East) that have a more balanced, accepting view of plastic surgery. It's something to be embraced rather than shunned.

As I discussed, the history of cosmetic enhancement dates back to Ancient Egypt, at least in recorded history, and is probably as old as time. Wanting to improve one's appearance and taking action to do so seems to be something that was important to human beings throughout history. Cosmetic surgery is embraced and celebrated by many cultures in the world today without the social condemnation or negative repercussions you see in America.

In later chapters, you'll see why your desire to look and feel better about yourself through cosmetic surgery should be guilt and shame-free, and is rooted in some very strong psychological, social, and even biological drives. But first, let's cover what may be an even bigger hurdle for you and your loved ones on your cosmetic surgery journey: the fear of something going wrong.

(3)

Fear: Why Does Plastic Surgery Go Wrong or Too Far?

Helping patients overcome their fears is a major part of my job. I am not there to sell, cajole, or coax anyone into doing anything they don't want to do. But I am there to counsel, advise, and deliver people from the "fear zone" and offer them a Transformational Experience™ that can change their lives in a profoundly positive way. People are scared, and rightly so. Having any work done is, let's face it, scary. So much uncertainty can make a potential plastic surgery patient paralyzed with fear.

Maybe fear is the main thing holding you back. What if something goes wrong? What will the outcome look like? Will it look unnatural or freakish? How do I know when I am taking it too far? In this chapter, we will talk about the fears you may be facing when considering plastic surgery.

WHAT IF...?

What if something goes wrong? All medical and surgical procedures carry a certain amount of risk, and cosmetic procedures are no different. There are general complications that can happen with almost any surgical procedure, such as infection, bleeding, poor healing, visible scarring, or even death. And then there are complications that are inherent to the specific cosmetic procedure, such as facial nerve injury with a facelift or double vision with a lower eyelid lift (blepharoplasty). While it is important to discuss specific risks with your surgeon for any procedure you are considering, dwelling on them can easily send you and your loved ones spiraling into the fear zone. If you find an excellent surgeon with good credentials (more on that later), serious complications or problems should be exceedingly rare. After all, this is cosmetic surgery, which means we care for healthy people with the goal of enhancing their appearance or making them better.

I think you'll agree that serious complications or problems **should be** exceedingly rare. I suggest you ask your prospective cosmetic surgeon or practitioner about any serious complications that may have happened in their practice. I am happy to report to my patients, in most cases, that I have never encountered the serious complication they are concerned about. Most complications in plastic surgery are not serious or permanent and can be addressed with proper care.

ADDRESSING FEARS: WILL I LIKE THE WAY I LOOK AFTERWARD? WHAT ABOUT DYING?

There are other ways things can go wrong beyond a serious complication, and you may just be fearful about how things will look when the dust settles and you are fully healed. What will the outcome look like? Despite the widespread availability of technology and imaging software that can show you how you will look after surgery, it should never be presented or seen as a guarantee of results or predictor of the outcome. There are a number of strategies that we will cover in a later chapter to make sure you choose the right doctor to get the specific outcome you desire. Using these strategies is your best way to overcome your fear and to ensure the ultimate success of your cosmetic procedure. Even the best surgeons have a certain percentage of patients who are unhappy with their outcomes. But at a certain point, you do have to put your trust and faith in that practitioner's skill.

Like a complication, a revision surgery or corrective cosmetic procedure should be something that is relatively rare in your doctor's experience with the procedure you are seeking. And you should again broach this subject with your prospective practitioner. Of course, I have the occasional revision in my practice, but it is always some minor tweak or improvement to something the patient was concerned about, never a major overhaul. If you go to a well-known surgeon with excellent credentials, this will almost always be the case with revisions of their own patients—performed in a very small percentage of cases.

What about the overwhelming fear that the outcome will be unnatural or freakish? We touched on this in the previous chapter, but if you ask the average American what they think about plastic surgery, the response is negative. Plastic, fake, phony, and botched. Celebrities who look nothing like their former selves permeate the American consciousness, and this gnawing fear is the first thing I hear when I meet prospective plastic surgery patients. "I don't want to look like [insert celebrity name here]." And the media, whether it is reality TV, the internet, or the tabloids, only serves to fuel this fear of plastic surgery. The favorite focus of these media outlets is on "plastic surgery nightmares." The "Catwoman," Donatella Versace, Joan Rivers, Michael Jackson, Mickey Rourke…the list goes on and on.

See image 1, again.

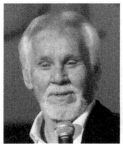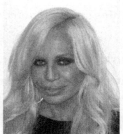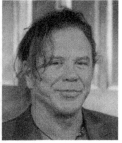

Left: Alamy photographer: Zuma. Center: Alamy photographer: dpa. Right: Alamy photographer: unknown

Endless pictures of people who bear little resemblance to their former selves through multiple, ill-conceived, and poorly executed plastic surgery procedures are pictured in the pages of the tabloids and their digital counterparts on the web.

Plastic surgery death, however uncommon, is another "nightmare" that is a favored focus. The death of Kanye West's mother during a liposuction and breast lift procedure received endless press. Plastic surgery deaths from extreme procedures, shady clinics, and medical tourism are all over the internet and tabloids.

When it comes to plastic surgery, our culture is hooked on the fantastic, the grotesque, and the dangerous elements of these medical procedures. This kind of information is featured most prominently on reality TV, the internet, and tabloids. Why is plastic surgery painted as such a three-ring circus? The short answer is because the drama sells. It gets our attention. Biologically speaking, the drama around plastic surgery activates our *amygdala*, which is part of our primitive, reptilian, or "lower brain" center. Collectively, these parts of our brain are called the *limbic system*. The limbic system is involved in our processing of emotions, including fear.

Our primitive brain or limbic system is constantly scanning our environment for danger. Once it senses something that could potentially be a threat, it sends signals to the rest of our brain and body—for example, hairs standing on end or heart racing that says, "Hey! There's something to pay attention to or to be afraid of here." For this reason, the news is heavily tilted toward what is going wrong with the world today instead of what is going right. We watch the negative stories on the news more attentively because we're thinking: "I need to know this there could be a threat here." This is the same reason reality TV, the internet, the tabloids, and the news focus more on the plastic surgery nightmares than on the everyday, run-of-the-mill success stories that are 99 percent of the reality of plastic surgery. The drama captures our attention more readily and is more interesting than the reality of these routine medical procedures. It's not surprising given the way that plastic surgery is portrayed in popular media that most Americans are scared to death to even consider having a procedure.

AVOIDING DISASTER

But beyond media sensationalism, a reasonable question in your mind may be "If celebrities have all the money and resources in the world, why the hell do celebrity disasters happen at all?" And, more importantly, "How do I keep a plastic surgery disaster from happening to me?"

So, what about *Botched* and celebrity disasters? The truth is, these kinds of cases constitute an extremely small percentage of plastic surgery cases. They capture our attention because we notice them. Like a bad accident we can't help but stare at, they capture our minds and highlight our fears. But the results that cause us to wonder, "What happened to that person's face, breasts, butt, etc.?" are the exception in plastic surgery, not the rule. There are a huge number of plastic surgery patients out there among you. You see them on the streets, in the stores, and on your movie screens, TV screens, and computers. They have results that are beautiful, natural, and undetectable. You don't notice them because, well, the results are *beautiful, natural, and undetectable.*

You may notice someone looks better than they used to, but you can't quite identify what they've done or what feature has been enhanced. Almost every celebrity or media personality past a certain age has had something done, from Botox to fillers to surgery. Do you think they just age better than the rest of us, coincidentally? Or maybe it's the night cream they are hocking on the Home Shopping Network? Having work done is much more commonplace in Hollywood than you would imagine, and it's unfortunate that the celebrity cases that are outliers are the only ones plastic surgery gets "credit" for.

Maybe you accept the premise that these cases of unnatural, noticeable, undesirable results are the rarity in plastic surgery and constitute a very small number of plastic surgery patients, but you're wondering why they happen at all. And why do they happen to celebrities who would go to the very best? It's because cosmetic enhancement is an elective procedure; it's a choice.

Cosmetic surgery is unlike other areas of medicine where if your symptoms are bad enough, you have no choice but to take medicine or have an operation. With cosmetic surgery, there is always a choice. Patients have a lot more power and say in what is done with cosmetic enhancement than in other areas of medicine or surgery. When having your thyroid removed, you would never ask the surgeon to take a little more off the left side than the right. But in the cosmetic surgery world, medicine is driven by the wants, needs, and desires of the patient because the success of the surgery or procedure is defined by patient satisfaction. While any board-certified cosmetic surgeon receives extensive training and education in what defines beauty, proportion, and a natural outcome, it doesn't mean achieving that end will satisfy the patient.

WHAT HAPPENED TO MICHAEL JACKSON'S NOSE AND JOAN RIVERS'S FACE?

So, what if the patient isn't satisfied? The patient had a procedure with a reasonable outcome, but they wanted something different. They may elect to have another pro-cedure with another surgeon and another outcome, and so on and so on. The plastic surgery nightmares you see in the media, on the internet, and in Hollywood are frequently the result of this vicious cycle.

What does everyone bring up when they think of a rhinoplasty or nose job? Michael Jackson. His case classically illustrates my point. Michael Jackson did not have one rhinoplasty; he had many. So many, in fact, that the exact number is a matter of speculation. Michael Jackson's first rhinoplasty was after the release of his fifth solo album, *Off the Wall*, in 1979. Jackson fell while dancing and broke his nose, and it's believed that's when he had his first plastic surgery. He actually had a very nice result. Here he is pictured with a slightly better, natural version of an ethnically appropriate African American nose. But after an untold number of rhinoplasties, the nose became deformed. The tissues could not handle repeated operations, blood flow was compromised, and tissue death even occurred in some areas. He ended up with what we in plastic surgery call an "end-stage nose" and a "nasal cripple." He had to resort to a prosthesis. Michael Jackson's nose was not the result of one or two surgeries with a few surgeons, but the result of multiple surgeries with multiple surgeons over a period of years.

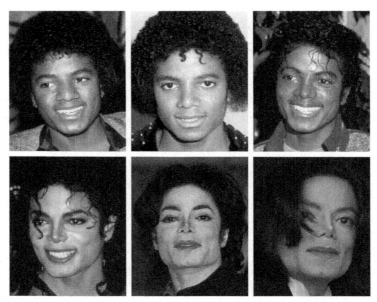

Top left: Alamy photographer: Pictorial Press. Top center: Alamy photographer: Mirrorpix. Top right: photographer unknown.

Bottom left: Alamy photographer: unknown. Bottom center: photographer: Interfoto/Personalities. Bottom right: Alamy photographer: Zuma

A result like this does not just happen. It is driven by the desire of the patient to achieve a certain outcome, which in the end is not realistic or achievable with plastic surgery. But clearly, some of the blame rests with surgeons who are willing to perform these operations. They're culpable not only technically, but also ethically. A surgeon must know when the risk of a poor or devastating outcome exceeds the benefit of operating. The surgeons in Michael Jackson's case did not know or care to accept their limits. Perhaps influenced by the power of celebrity or the financial gain that comes with operating on the ultimate celebrity, they, through arrogance or hubris, convinced themselves they could be a hero, but it had devastating consequences.

How about celebrity facelifts gone wrong? What celebrity comes to mind? Joan Rivers. A lot of facelift patients say they don't want to look like her. Overly pulled, overly stuffed, and not quite looking like the youthful Joan of the 1980s with a thinner, gaunter face.

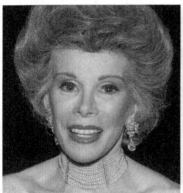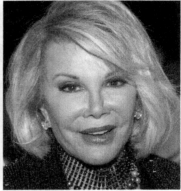

Left: Alamy photographer: Media Punch. Right: Alamy stock photo/contributor: Steve Mack

In her case, intention was the key. It was reported by her daughter Melissa in the memoir *The Book of Joan: Tales of Mirth, Mischief, and Manipulation* that Joan had an unimaginable 348 cosmetic operations over the course of her lifetime. Rivers never shied away from speaking openly and unabashedly about her plastic surgery and her addiction to it. She never felt pretty and felt she had a thin face and homely features. Intentionally over many years, she had many operations, and many surgeons sought to change the way she originally looked. Her love for plastic surgery was the subject of many of her jokes: "Every weekend I just go in, and I do something new. I get a tenth one free. It's a little like coffee. You just keep going." And I can't help but include this joke: "I have had so much plastic surgery, when I die they will donate my body to Tupperware."

Perhaps one of the most horrific celebrity examples of the vicious cycle of repeated operations is Jocelyn Wildenstein, or as people call her, "Catwoman."

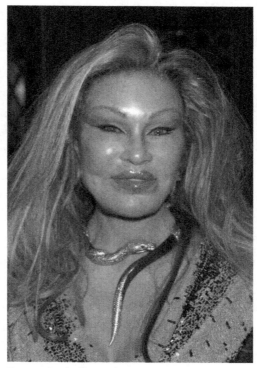

Shutterstock: s_buckley

It's reported that Wildenstein spent millions of dollars on plastic surgery to please her cat-loving, art-dealing husband, Alec Wildenstein. She had a number of procedures including an operation called a *canthoplasty*, which was done in an overly aggressive manner to create the slanted eyes of a cat.

Jocelyn Wildenstein first became known after her highly public divorce from billionaire art dealer Alec Wildenstein in 1999. In a record-breaking settlement for that year, she took home roughly $2.5 billion. Her estranged husband, Alec, died in 2008. Strangely, she denies having had any plastic surgery, and she credits her Swiss heritage for her high cheekbones and exaggerated features. Again, the key here was a patient who had an intention for a certain look with pulled eyes and overstuffed lips and face, and who cycled through many procedures and surgeons to end up looking like a lioness.

My point in discussing these celebrity examples is not to be salacious or controversial, but to squarely address the false impression and fear that many people have, especially those new to considering cosmetic work. They're afraid they will somehow end up looking like one of these celebrities after the work is done and the bandages are removed. Those kinds of results do not happen suddenly and by accident. They are the result of many operations over many years, with many different surgeons; and they are driven by the unrealistic wants, needs, and desires of the celebrities seeking them.

If you approach cosmetic surgery with reasonable expectations for improvement and seek out an excellent surgeon by following the steps outlined in the upcoming chapters, plastic surgery can and will deliver the natural, life-changing results you are looking for. There is little to no chance you will end up like one of these celebrity nightmares.

WHAT IF I TAKE IT TOO FAR?

Lastly, a common fear that potential plastic surgery patients have—and that you may have—is you will either become "addicted" to plastic surgery or just plain go overboard. So how do you know as a plastic surgery patient, or as the loved one of a patient, when you or your loved one are "taking things too far"?

As we will see in the upcoming chapters, our physical appearance influences our social interactions and success in life much more than perhaps you ever thought possible. After reading this book, you will feel good about your decision to pursue cosmetic enhancement, and as the title says, you won't "(Don't) feel bad about looking good." You will find optimizing your appearance to be a smart, life-affirming choice. But, of course, as with all things in life, there can be a healthy attitude toward this process, and there can be a point where it becomes an obsession.

Obsession or addiction are not unique to cosmetic surgery

or cosmetic enhancement, although unhealthy obsession or vanity appears to be the first thing people are accused of when they even broach the subject of plastic surgery with their friends or loved ones. All things in life have a point where they cross the line from healthy to harmful if done in excess. Even exercise, if done to the extreme, can cause immense physical harm to the body. No one would accuse someone who exercises once a day of an unhealthy obsession. Yet one visit to the cosmetic surgeon's office and your friends and family may land you in the nutty bin. We covered in detail in earlier chapters why a generally negative opinion exists regarding plastic surgery, but even if you are pursuing it the right way and in moderation, with fantastic, natural results, you will face your fair share of naysayers and haters. But if someone accuses you of being cosmetic surgery obsessed, how do you know when they may be right?

Knowing the difference between someone with a healthy attitude toward cosmetic enhancement and someone who is taking it too far, and albeit rare, a person who is mentally ill, is another key skill that I must employ in every interaction I have with a patient. I use this skill every time I see someone, and on some days, that means sixty or seventy times a day.

I've really had to sharpen this skill; it's to the point where it is almost a sixth sense. "Can I make this person happy (with this procedure)?" I ask myself. "Is what they are asking for realistic?" If the answer to either of these questions is "No,

I can't," then I won't do what the patient is asking. This is my red line, my sine qua non. As a physician, I take the ethical charge of "do no harm" very seriously. I couldn't sleep at night if I didn't. To me, performing a procedure that has risks, won't satisfy a patient's needs, and costs money, is doing harm. My job is to keep people safe and make them happy.

Based on my description, it probably sounds like this is easy and I have a handle on it. But if you ask anyone who does what I do for a living, they'll tell you the most challenging part of our job is dealing with people. As technically challenging as the procedures are, as grueling as the schedule is, and as difficult as it is to keep up in a field that evolves at breakneck speed, nothing is harder for a cosmetic surgeon than knowing when to operate or perform a procedure, and when to say no. Nothing hurts us to the core more than when we have failed to satisfy a patient's needs or operated on the "wrong patient" (a patient we can't satisfy).

After all, what kind of people do you think become cosmetic surgeons? Type-A perfectionists who think: "Hell, I can take apart that person's face and make it look better." What do you think a type-A perfectionists want to avoid the most? A mistake, or even the perception of a mistake. And in cosmetic surgery, mistakes or perceived errors are as plain as the nose on your face, pun intended.

Baseball players get multimillion-dollar contracts for hitting the ball one in three times. CEOs get golden parachutes for bankrupting companies, and in your own job, a mistake, even a big one, may not be the end of the world. My life as a facial plastic surgeon is a zero-tolerance game. What makes it tougher for our type-A personalities is accepting that the definition of "getting it right" can be completely out of our control. I have sometimes performed technically perfect surgeries with an aesthetically ideal outcome, yet had a raving-mad patient. Other times I misread a person. I have at other times, despite all my technical and psychological skills developed over the past twenty years, operated on the wrong patient (someone I could never satisfy). These are the cases that keep surgeons up at night.

Sadly, I sometimes struggle to focus on the tens of thousands of people I have made happy, and I'm kept awake thinking about the small number of patients who are less than thrilled or downright unhappy. How do I know it's such a small number? I keep statistics. But just like a product on Amazon, I have a near five-star rating and more Google reviews than many other cosmetic surgeons in New York. I am in the top 1 percent of cosmetic surgery providers in the United States, but I am tormented by the few patients I have not made happy. And these patients are free to vent their unhappiness and criticisms, whether fair or unfair, on the internet for the entire world to see. I am in a zero-tolerance field with no room to be, well, human.

BODY DYSMORPHIC DISORDER

I do not confess the above for sympathy. After all, I chose this field even if the reality of its perfectionism never really hit me when I was in training. I confess the above to let you know how motivated I am both to "do no harm" (or in my case, "only do perfect") through my ethical charge as a physician and surgeon, but to avoid, as much as humanly possible, cases that make me feel like a failure. Even with this intense drive and motivation, I get it wrong sometimes, and so does anyone else who does what I do for a living. Why? It's because human beings are complex. There are psychological screening tools to help detect Body Dysmorphic Disorder (BDD). An excellent test and one that is fairly accurate for assessing the mental state of plastic surgery and dermatology patients is the Body Dysmorphic Disorder Questionnaire (BDDQ). In practice and application, however, the test is not that helpful. Imagine me having to say to my patient, "Um...hold on...I would like you to complete this questionnaire because I suspect you might have a mental illness."

While the exact percentage of cosmetic surgery patients who have BDD is not clear (studies estimate it's between 2 and 10 percent), we know these patients represent a small fraction of those pursuing cosmetic surgery. In other words, you are not vain, you are not obsessed, and at least 90 to 98 percent of you are not psychologically ill because you are pursuing cosmetic surgery or enhancement. So, ignore the naysayers and haters. But how do we know when we or a loved one are potentially crossing the line with cosmetic surgery or enhancement? This question is much more difficult to answer than it seems at face value, as you will see in a moment. Admittedly, I do not have all the answers in regard to this question.

To repeat, human beings are complex. But clearly, when a patient exhibits signs and symptoms of Body Dysmorphic Disorder, a surgeon and patient should not cross that line. So, how do mental-health professionals know when someone has BDD? They consult the manual: the DSM-5, which is the *Diagnostic and Statistical Manual, Fifth Version*. This is the compendium of mental illness and personality disorders that psychiatrists use to diagnose a patient.

For someone to be diagnosed with BDD they must meet four criteria: (1) preoccupation with appearance; (2) exhibit repetitive (compulsive) behavior (e.g., mirror checking, excessive grooming, skin picking); (3) clinical significance (i.e., their preoccupation must impair their ability to function socially or occupationally); (4) differentiation from an eating disorder (i.e., their preoccupation is not with their weight).

BDD is listed under the category of Obsessive Compulsive Disorder (OCD). Much like OCD patients, BBD patients are plagued with unrelenting compulsive thoughts that dominate their thinking and ruin their life. In BDD, the thoughts just happen to be related to a physical flaw, rather than something else. If someone exhibits signs and symptoms of BDD, they clearly should not have cosmetic work done and should be referred for psychological evaluation and treatment.

For a patient with BDD, having a procedure never relieves their obsession with the real or perceived flaw, and in some cases can make the illness worse. Once a procedure is performed, the focus of a BDD patient's obsession may change, but the obsessive thoughts and patterns will still be there. For example, a person with BDD has a nose job because they feel their nose is too big for their face, and once their nose is smaller they find another flaw to focus on, such as their chin. When undetected, BDD patients go from doctor to doctor in an attempt to relieve their obsession. They may have multiple unnecessary procedures, and in the worst cases, they end up disfigured.

I have encountered quite a few patients with BDD. In any patient evaluation, I scan for clues to identify those who have this disorder. Even the patients with the mildest forms of BDD are pretty intense and intent. The emotional intensity they communicate through their speech and body language regarding their area of concern is beyond that of the standard patient. This intensity and focus is so palpable in the conversation, it immediately tips me off that I may be dealing with a BDD patient. Since patients with BDD can have a "perceived" flaw, it's obvious to me the patient may have a psychological problem when I don't see the same thing they do.

These kinds of patients are the easiest to spot. For example, they may complain their chin is weak, when they actually have a chin and jawline that could cut through butter. Or a flaw may be present, but not to the degree perceived. For example, someone may say, "I have the worst nose ever," when in fact, they have an attractive nose with maybe a slight but attractive bump. BDD patients are the first to grab mirrors, point to their flaws, and demand I see the same thing they do. They come in with a myriad of pictures on their cell phones from different angles with different lighting. They show me how bad the problem is and demand for me to make them look the same from every angle with different lighting, which is a physical impossibility. They bring in pictures of other people: real people, celebrities, and anyone else they would rather look like. Then, they ask me to transform them into anyone but themselves.

While BDD patients may have one perceived flaw, most don't, and the topic of conversation can easily change from how they're unhappy with their nose to how they're unhappy about their chin, and then they talk about their hairline, while those features are either perfect or as good as they could be.

Also, BDD patients usually reveal that they are "doctor hoppers." They may have had a few procedures done on different body parts already. They are clearly unhappy or less than satisfied with the work, and they blame it on the doctor's lack of skill or unwillingness to do what they wanted. However, the work they've had is quite good or as good as could be expected.

When I encounter a patient like this, I listen and I am supportive. Confrontation with "reality" does not work. To suggest what they see is not real or less than what they perceive would only be met with rapid indignation and rebuttal. Referral for psychological or psychiatric counseling is the most appropriate course of action for a physician encountering such a patient, but this is a lot easier in theory than in practice. Broaching the subject that they may have a mental illness, as you could imagine, does not go well with a BDD patient. As is the case with most mental illnesses, they are not self-aware. I'm explaining BDD and the symptoms you might see to help you better identify when you or a loved one may be crossing a line into the pathological when seeking cosmetic services. The sad part is, if you have BDD and you are reading this, you probably won't realize it.

INFLUENCE OF THE DIGITAL AGE

As we discussed, a small minority of patients seeking cosmetic surgery fit the criterion for a clinical diagnosis of BDD.

But, let me repeat, human beings are complex. BDD is not black and white in that you either have it or you don't. I think everyone can exhibit obsessive behaviors with regard to a particular body part or trait, even in the absence of full-blown BDD. This makes the choice for me to operate or not to operate, to inject or not to inject, more complex today than it ever has been. Why? You probably guessed it: the digital age. We see ourselves a hell of a lot more than people did ten or even twenty years ago. What changed? Social media posts, selfies, Instagram, Snapchat, filters, and Facetune, that's what!

The facility, dependence, and obsession of multiple generations (Millennial, Gen Z, Gen Alpha) with social media and digital images of themselves has exploded. Before digital cameras, who the hell would ever think of taking a picture of themselves? But today, selfies are part of our culture. Patients confront me with these selfies—pictures taken at various angles with different lighting—and when their appearance doesn't match the perfect, filtered features they see in their social media posts, I am asked to "fix the problem." Millennials and younger generations are flocking to cosmetic surgery offices in equal numbers as baby boomers. According to the 2018 American Academy of Facial Plastic Surgery annual survey, 72 percent of facial plastic surgeons have seen an increase in patients under the age of thirty!

I see more and more people in their twenties and even teens

with near-perfect features and no signs of aging. They ask for fillers to enhance their jawline or Botox to prevent their wrinkles. Are these new generations more vain? No, they are just focused on social media and how they appear to others through their posts. The social advantage garnered by their appearance is instantaneously seen on their phones by the number of Instagram likes or Snapchat. They are more focused on their personal image because of the rapidity of feedback they receive. The dopamine rushes they get from many likes or views can almost have an addictive property, and we see this addiction with many of the younger generations—their faces are constantly buried in their phones. In fact, repetitively checking the phone for this feedback can cross over into the obsessive-compulsive spectrum. While these cases are clearly far afield from someone with BDD, I bring them up to illustrate that the decision whether or not to intervene becomes much more of a blurred line.

Intervening in these cases of social media obsessed kids in their teens and twenties is more about enhancing an already normal feature, and much less like my usual work of fixing a feature that is less than attractive, or a defect. This kind of intervention has become more commonplace in my work. And to be completely honest, I do feel a bit more uncomfortable and uncertain of myself ethically when it comes to approaching a patient who would like to be "better than normal." But really, when it comes down to it, my work is about making people happier with the way they look. As long as I can do it safely and do no harm, it is not my place to judge a patient's decision to spend their money and effort to conform to their own ideal. I know if I were to turn these patients down, they would just end up in someone else's office who perhaps wouldn't be as safe or conservative with their recommendations.

IS THERE A "DO NOT CROSS" LINE? WHAT IF SOMEONE ALREADY WENT TOO FAR?

There are also cases where I'm asked to go beyond enhancement to create a look I don't necessarily feel is natural or attractive. Where do I draw the line? The line, at least for me, is this: If I feel the results are not aiming toward a more aesthetic or beautiful outcome, if I feel the results would create a disproportion or natural imbalance, or if it just doesn't make sense to do what the patient is asking, then I politely explain to the patient why I won't do the procedure. Most patients will appreciate my honesty and aesthetic judgment because I do this for a living. Others, I'm sure, are disappointed and will maybe go elsewhere. At the end of the day, though, every face and every feature I work on is, in part, my calling card. Patients will and do talk to others about where they've had work done, and who did the work, so of course, I would like others to have a favorable impression of my life's work.

If you were to spend some time in my waiting room, a huge

percentage of the people you will see have normal, natural, undetectable results. It may not even be clear to you exactly what work they've had done. To be completely honest, however, there are some patients who might scare the hell out of you. Sometimes, they scare the hell out of other prospective patients, who say to me: "I saw this patient in the waiting room and I thought, 'I hope you didn't do that!'" I cringe and, of course, want to scream a resounding: "No!"

Since patients talk about the work they've had done, it's less than ideal when I do "work" on top of previous work. This is because the minute I touch them, they tell their friends that I am their doctor, and I am damned by association. Even though I don't agree with the aesthetic choices the patient or their previous surgeon or surgeons have made, I don't turn those patients away. Revision, corrective surgery, or helping tweak a patient who wants something more even after what I consider to be bad work is part of my job, and it's my chance to help someone. It comes with the territory. The chance to help is more important than the risk of guilt by association.

In this chapter, we tackled some of the most common fears people face when considering cosmetic surgery. These fears can be paralyzing and prevent people from ever making the change they want to make. These fears are typically echoed by those closest to them when they confide in them about considering plastic surgery or a non-surgical procedure. We addressed the fear of complications and how they are relatively uncommon in the world of cosmetic enhance-ment. We talked about the fear of the unknown and how anxiety over the outcome of the procedure can be reduced by selecting a good surgeon with a low revision rate. We tackled the question on almost everyone's mind regarding plastic surgery and explained how celebrity disasters occur. The plastic surgery nightmares that dominate the American consciousness don't just happen by a slip of the syringe or the knife. As made obvious from the celebrity nightmares we discussed, these kinds of outcomes are the exception rather than the rule. They will not happen to you if you do your research, find a qualified surgeon, research his or her results, have an eye toward improvement rather than per-fection, and want to be natural, not ubernatural. Overdone, overexaggerated plastic surgery outcomes are conscious (or sometimes unconscious) choices caused by patient drive as much as surgeon skill or lack thereof.

We talked about the fear of becoming "addicted" to plastic surgery. As you can see from our discussion in this chap-ter, the choice to have a procedure (or two, or ten) does not make you a plastic surgery junkie. We talked about a healthy attitude toward plastic surgery and how to identify when you or someone you know might be taking it too far. The social media age we live in has perhaps heightened the risk for both the younger and older generations to seek filtered results, or seek the features of another person, which may not be entirely achievable with plastic surgery.

We learned a bit about Body Dysmorphic Disorder and that it is relatively rare in patients seeking plastic surgical enhancement. We learned how to spot the signs and why these patients should not have procedures, but instead be referred for psychological counseling. I shared the choices I face with patients every day, and understanding the decision of whether or not to perform a procedure is becoming increasingly blurred for surgeons who try to "do no harm" and follow their ethical charge. When you find a surgeon you connect with who is qualified, ethical, and achieves natural outcomes, my best advice is to listen to their guidance if they tell you they cannot achieve the kind of result you are looking for.

To recap the first three chapters, we discussed a lot about the negative energy surrounding plastic surgery and anti-aging aesthetic medicine. Guilt, shame, and fear are emotions every patient faces in their journey to transform their lives through plastic surgery or non-surgical procedures. Guilt, shame, and fear can make people feel bad about wanting to look good. But there are plenty of reasons to feel good about your decision to look and feel your best, and to take advantage of the advances medical science has to offer. In the following chapters, we'll explore why you shouldn't feel bad about wanting to look your best.

The Connection between Looking and Feeling Good

There is an undeniable connection between how we look and how we feel. I don't think I could have said it any better than one of my patients: "I think one always has that thought [guilt] crop up. The expense, time off of work, alternate uses for the money...all of these play a part. But, as I tell others, 'You spend money on your car, oil changes, new mufflers, and paint jobs. Why would you take any less care of yourself?' I'm a big fan of caring for the physical, emotional, and energetic aspects of oneself! All deserve love and attention! I am a Holistic Practitioner, and I know the link between our physical and emotional health. These two are interconnected. When we feel that we look our best, that translates internally to augment our feelings of confidence and vitality.

The two aspects, physical and emotional, work to support one another and form the picture of who we perceive ourselves to be."

THE OUTSIDE REFLECTS THE INSIDE AND VICE VERSA

How we look affects how we feel about ourselves, and it impacts our interactions with others and the world around us to a greater degree than most would admit. Think back to being a teenager. Did you ever have a pimple or a monster zit for the whole world to see? Was it so big that you wanted to hide your face? Did it affect your confidence that day? Did you engage with others and engage in life as much when you felt the whole world was staring at this disgusting thing on your face? Probably not. You probably felt self-conscious. Maybe you didn't talk to your friends as much, and you definitely avoided engaging with any potential romantic interests. Maybe you declined a couple of dates until after it was gone. When your skin cleared up, your self-confidence miraculously returned. You felt lighter and willing to see and be seen. What if you were more unfortunate with your skin and had more than the occasional outbreak, but constant cystic acne? Millions of people do. Then, instead of having periods of clear skin, your skin was always embarrassing, always affecting how you looked and felt about yourself. I'm sure we can all relate to these stories, as not many people escape adolescence without at least the occasional pimple that made them want to stick their faces in the sand.

Yes, we might be a little more self-conscious in adolescence than we are as adults, but the truth of the matter is *we all care*. Our brains are programmed to care. Our brains are also programmed to care about how other people look. This is easy to see from the pimple discussion, and I apologize if this example conjured up painful memories. I highlighted this to illustrate how easily a physical flaw or perceived physical flaw can have a profound psychological impact on us. The bottom line is we cannot separate how we look from how we feel. Why does how we look have such an impact on our psychological well-being? Are we being vain by caring what we look like? No. I would argue that we are being human.

DEVELOPING OUR SELF-IMAGE

As humans, the very notion of who we are, our so-called "self-image," develops from birth and is formed to a great degree not only by our visual perception of ourselves, but from the feedback we get about our appearance from the world around us. As strange as it may seem, visual perception and self-judgment come second in both timing and importance in forming our self-image. Of course, infants don't really have access to mirrors before they start walking, so they rarely see their own faces except for in the occasional mirror included in a walker, mobile, or toy. It doesn't matter much anyway, because we don't even recognize our own reflection until about the age of two.

A study in the journal *Developmental Psychobiology*[5] sought to determine when the first indication of self-image or awareness was present in children from the ages of three months to twenty-four months by observing their behavior in front of a mirror. Infants at first largely ignore their mirror reflections. The first prolonged and repeated reaction of an infant to his mirror image is that of a sociable "playmate" from about six through twelve months of age. In other words, just like a dog that barks at herself in the mirror, infants don't know their own reflection; they think it is another child to interact with. In the second year of life, children begin to recognize their image as their own and exhibit wariness and withdrawal from their reflection. Of course, self-admiration also accompanied those behaviors starting at fourteen months and was demonstrated by 75 percent of the subjects after twenty months of age. Beyond that age, the typical fascination we have for ourselves finally takes hold, and we not only recognize ourselves but begin to "ham it up" and test out different facial expressions and poses. However, our self-image develops much earlier than the age of two, before we have the ability to recognize our own face in the mirror.

Self-image begins forming at birth. Of course, the earliest input we get is from our parents. The "ooing" and "ahhing" in infancy, hopefully from loving parents, helps to create a

5   "Mirror Self-Image Reactions before Age Two," *Developmental Psychobiology* 5, no. 4 (1972): 297–305.

positive self-image or basis for most of us. Parents and siblings are the first to give us feedback on our appearance, but we get plenty of input from others in every social interaction we have. And nowhere do people feel more comfortable than offering input on physical image or appearance than with babies or children. "Oh, he looks just like his mother," "Look at those freckles," "Look at those big cheeks!" "She's pretty," "She's tall, just like her father," "What a cute little kid!" Could you imagine us going around making those kinds of comments as adults to people we just met? Somehow with babies or children, a running commentary on physical traits is more acceptable and even invited by parents.

Of course, there is also less flattering input one may hear from the brash, drunk uncle or from kids on the playground: "Look at those big ears; it's Dumbo, junior!" "He has his father's nose" (translated: big beak), "She's very *interesting* looking" (i.e., homely). Nowhere is our attention more rapt than when others are talking or commenting about us. We take in these statements, both good and bad, combine them with our own perceived image, and form a composite self-image. Statements like "I am fat," "I am beautiful," "I am short," "I am smart," become ingrained in both our conscious and subconscious mind to form a complete mental picture of who we are.

Our self-image becomes a series of beliefs we hold to be "true" about ourselves. A person's self-image influences greatly how they feel about themselves as well as every social interaction they have. While most of our self-image is formed by late adolescence, it's not completely static or inelastic throughout our lives. People change throughout their lives, and their view of themselves can certainly change as well. Yet, what we have to understand is that our view of ourselves, how we feel about how we look, and who we are was not formed in a vacuum, and does not exist in a vacuum. It is hugely influenced by the feedback we get from others around us.

TO BE HUMAN IS TO BE VISUAL AND SOCIAL

Human beings are intensely visual and social creatures. In the brain itself, there are hundreds of millions of neurons (brain cells) devoted to visual processing. Neurons dedicated to vision make up about 30 percent of the cortex, as compared to only 8 percent for touch and 3 percent for hearing. Each of the two optic nerves, which carry signals from the retina to the brain, consist of a million fibers, while each auditory nerve carries a mere thirty thousand. We learn much faster and remember much better when the information we receive from the world is presented visually rather than verbally.

Our brains are constantly scanning the environment for visual input. A team of neuroscientists from MIT found that the human brain can process entire images the eyes see in as little as thirteen milliseconds. The digestion of information is so rapid, it's almost entirely on a subconscious level. It makes sense that our brain dedicates so much processing power to visual information, because it's the most abundant and rapid source of information we are exposed to.

Why is it so important for us to gather information about our environment quickly and efficiently? Because our very survival depends on it. Evolutionarily, if we were to rely on another way of getting information, we would not have survived for very long. Imagine a saber-toothed tiger approaching our ancestors. Instead of relying upon sight, what if they attempted to hear the tiger or smell him approaching to avoid being devoured? How would that have worked out for them? Of course, this very ridiculous example highlights that we are visual beings, and our brains are visually biased, environment-scanning machines.

Humans are intensely visual evolutionarily, but also intensely social. We form social bonds from the moment we are born. A large part of our brain is dedicated to processing social information. The striatum and other brain sites including the amygdala, ventromedial prefrontal cortex, and lateral prefrontal cortex all play a role in reward processing and social behavior. Activity in these brain networks allows for flexible changes in evaluation of stimuli from the social world. In fact, these social centers are so developed in the human brain that scientists have posited the "social brain theory" to explain the vast differences between the human brain and that of other species. The brain size of the great ape species closest in evolution to humans (such as chimpanzees and bonobos) is only 25 to 35 percent of modern human brain size. The "social brain theory" states that our larger brain size is explained mostly, or at least in part, by our more sophisticated social bonds and interactions.

Further evidence of this theory is apparent in the way the human brain grows. The newborn human brain is only 25 percent of its adult volume as opposed to 50–70 percent in newborn apes. The rapid growth of the human brain in the first few years of life corresponds to the period of most rapid social development. We form families, tribes, cities, countries, and relate to the world around us through the prism of our social network. Being "social" is so important to the human brain that most psychological illnesses (i.e., brain malfunctions) are defined at least in part by how the illness affects our relation to others. One of the hallmarks for depression, for example, is decreased social interaction or social isolation. On the contrary, someone with a healthy, well-adjusted brain is engaged with others and has meaningful relationships.

Being visual and being social defines what it means to be, well, human. We receive, process, react to, and give great importance to social information we receive visually. We cannot deny these essential facets of the human brain borne by science and millions of years of evolution.

THE IMPORTANCE OF FACES

From the moment we are born, the most important social information and the information the baby brain focuses on is visual—in particular, another person's face. Watch a baby's eyes scan up and down anyone's face that comes close to it. The baby is absorbing millions of pieces of information synthesized automatically, instantly, and subconsciously by the very new and moldable human brain. The human brain has a facial recognition center whose sole purpose is to memorize and record features of the human face for rapid recall. It is called the fusiform face area (FFA), and it's a region of the ventral temporal cortex in the fusiform gyrus, which is an area in the temporal lobe that is believed to be necessary for facial recognition.

Why might dedicating an entire center of the brain to facial recall be important from a survival standpoint? Well, for example, it's important to recognize your mom's face, who provides your sole means of sustenance in the early months before you can even hold your head up. Or, to recognize your father's face, who may provide some protection from animals or others who may attempt to harm you in the defenseless newborn state. And you may want to help your parents to remember your face by activating their FFA (fusiform face area) with some fun visual social cues like a big smile, for example. So, we relate to each other visually through our facial expressions from the moment of birth.

As we discussed, facial recognition is pretty important, but there is other critical information we receive from faces that we relate to visually and integrate socially. Some of the most important information conveyed by the human face is emotion. The human face has forty-three muscles capable of creating a multitude of expressions. These facial expressions can instantaneously signal a wealth of information. Scientists from Ohio State University counted at least twenty-one different facial expressions and were able to map those consistently to be recognized in computer algorithms.[6]

Activation of specific facial muscles conveys and communicates our emotional state to others. For example, contraction of the zygomaticus major muscle raises the corners of our mouth and signals happiness. Contraction of our corrugator and procerus muscles between our brows, along with activation of the depressor anguli oris muscle, sends the message, "I'm really pissed off." Our brains understand these expressions to convey certain emotions even before we are capable of spoken language. Interpretation of visual cues from faces happens so rapidly in the brain that it's at the subconscious level.

How might the rapid transmission of emotional informa-

6   Ramprakash Srinivasan, Julie D. Golomb, and Aleix M. Martinez, "A Neural Basis of Facial
    Action Recognition in Humans," *Journal of Neuroscience* 36, no. 16 (2016): 4434–42; DOI:
    https://doi.org/10.1523/JNEUROSCI.1704-15.2016.

tion through facial expressions have been important to our survival evolutionarily? Well, you may not have wanted to approach your tribal chief around the campfire when his brow was furrowed, and his nasal muscles were flaring, because it may have cost you your life. Thinking more positively, a smile returned in kind might have signaled that it was time for you to make your move on a potential mate. Picking up on others' facial cues is clearly a critical aspect of human communication. It has been estimated that 93 percent of communication is nonverbal, with 55 percent of that coming from visual cues.[7,8,9,10] Visual communication is so important in conveying our emotional state that we've even invented emojis to supplement simple texts that can't capture what we're feeling.

Here's a modern-day example to further illustrate the importance of visual cues in communication. My son and I were recently eating at a local establishment that was one of the first to offer "bubble tea," the tea with edible boba pearls made of tapioca. We like bubble tea, so we happened to go twice in a single week. Behind the counter was a pleasant young gentleman who didn't say much to us other than transactional phrases like "Here's your credit card, Sir."

7   A. Mehrabian and M. Wiener, "Decoding of Inconsistent Communications," *Journal of Personality and Social Psychology* 6 (1967): 109–14.

8   A. Mehrabian and S. R. Ferris, "Inference of Attitudes from Nonverbal Communication in Two Channels," *Journal of Consulting Psychology* 31, no. 3 (1967): 48–258.

9   A. Mehrabian, *Silent Messages* (Wadsworth, CA: Belmont, 1971).

10 A. Mehrabian, *Nonverbal Communication* (Chicago: Aldine-Atherton, 1972).

Yet he always wore the biggest, warmest smile on his face while he was helping with our order. As we got in the car, my son and I said almost simultaneously: "Nice guy. Do you think he's the owner?" Now, why would we both think he's the owner of the place? He barely said anything to us. It's because we interpreted his nonverbal communication to say, "I care about you guys as customers, and I care about this place." Visual, nonverbal communication is sometimes much more important than the words we say. People can see what we believe is kept in our own internal, private world, but it's literally "written" all over our faces.

Beyond recognizing someone's face or figuring out what their emotional state may be, our brains are also "hardwired" to make judgments about the attractiveness, or conversely, the repulsiveness, of another person's face. Sounds harsh, doesn't it? But that is exactly what we do, or should I say, what our brains do, as human beings. This evaluation and judgment of faces happens rapidly and subconsciously. It is instinctual, present from birth, and, you guessed it, has roots in our evolution as visual and social beings.

As human beings, we all have a natural preference for attractive faces. But how do we all know what the definition of "attractive" is? After all, isn't beauty in the eye of the beholder? No, not really. Psychological research shows the most attractive human face is one that doesn't appear to be striking. It's not the exotic face, but strangely enough, the average one. Studies have shown that faces become more attractive when computer morphing (face-changing) software is used to blend or distort to create an average face.[11,12] This predilection toward average or attractive faces seems to be "hardwired" and present from birth.

Research conducted by Alan Slater from the University of Exeter in the UK showed that even newborns exhibit a distinct gaze preference toward more attractive faces. This hardwired judgment continues into adulthood. Multiple studies have also shown that unattractive infant faces may elicit negative facial expressions from adults. Attractiveness influences how adults interact with children, which ultimately has a major effect on the infant's personality and development.[13,14] We naturally shun what we deem to be unattractive. We shun anything outside of the norm, especially when it comes to the face.

Throughout history, people born with facial birth defects have been shunned, abandoned, or even killed. African tribes prohibited anyone with a facial irregularity from

---

11   J. H. Langlois, L. A. Roggman, "Attractive Faces Are Only Average, *Psychological Science* (1990), journals.sagepub.com

12   Gillian Rhodes and Tanya Tremewan, "Averageness, Exaggeration, and Facial Attractiveness," first published March 1, 1996, research article, *Psychological Science*; DOI: https://doi.org/10.1111/j.1467-9280.1996.tb00338.x.

13   S. S. Schein and J. H. Langlois, "Unattractive Infant Faces Elicit Negative Affect from Adults," *Infant Behavior and Development* 38 (2015): 130–34; DOI: 10.1016/j.infbeh.2014.12.009.

14   C. W. Stephan and J. H. Langlois, "Baby Beautiful: Adult Attributions of Infant Competence as a Function of Infant Attractiveness," *Child Development* 55 (1984): 576–85.

being elevated to chief. In India, families with a child who had a deformity were cast into the lower social class. In Ancient Rome, facial deformities were seen as a curse from the gods, and deformed babies were sacrificed out of fear. Studies show that even in modern times, people born with birth defects are severely stigmatized by other children and adults, and they suffer serious psychosocial consequences in everyday life.[15] When we see someone with anything "wrong" with their face—for example, a deformity, a burn, big eye bags, sunken cheeks, or even bad wrinkles—the truth is we cannot help but stare as we try to interpret the situation. We get a strange sense that we should avoid interaction. When we see someone with an attractive or, as we learned, strikingly average face, we might also stare, but usually with the opposite vibe. We are attracted to and sympathetic toward the beautiful face. Are we just being cruel, vapid humans, treating others as objects for our fascination and judgment? The answer is no. This is hardwired in our brains.

So why do our brains think it is so important to make judgments about other people's faces that it's a hardwired function present from birth? Because during evolution, our continued existence may have required this skill. Judgments about the human face can convey information about the relative health or disease of another person. Many communicable illnesses (e.g., syphilis, leprosy, or tuberculosis,

15 W. C. Shaw, "Folklore Surrounding Facial Deformity and the Origins of Facial Prejudice," *British Journal of Plastic Surgery* 34 (1981): 237–46.

to name just a few) can lead to facial flaws or even facial deformities. Our aversion to people with something out of place on their face is not due to morbid fascination, but it serves as a signal to us: "Hey, I'd better stay away from that person. They may have something I can catch."

Beyond an indicator of illness, evaluating a person's face may be a way of "reading" their genes. Many facial deformities are associated with other serious genetic errors, making survival and procreation much less likely in the harsh world of primitive man. Conversely, a perfect face with no flaws conveys by the law of averages good genes and stock to pass on to the next generation. Eye bags, wrinkles, a receding hairline, and other signs of facial aging are correctly associated with "aging genes" and can be telltale signs of illness. Even now that our survival doesn't necessarily depend on this identification and we have more information regarding health and disease, our brains still make these snap judgments for us. By nature, we judge people's faces as healthy or unhealthy, or as attractive or repulsive.

Our physical appearance affects how we feel about ourselves, not only through our own perception, but through the feedback we receive from others around us. Like it or not, the human brain is a visual/social judgment machine. Think about a time in your adult life when you attended a large gathering of people like a party, a school function, or a large meeting. What is your brain largely engaged in doing while you sit or stand waiting for things to start? You are visually scanning the crowd. Your brain is instantaneously gathering millions of bits of information about what others look like and what it might mean. Think about the comments you make to your closest confidants after such an event: "Wow, did you see Joe? He lost a lot of weight!" "Francesca looked great with her new haircut," "Tom lost a lot of hair..." and so on.

Whether we like it or not, human beings are visual and social. You can deny this evolutionary reality and think we have evolved beyond such superficial considerations and view someone more deeply: their soul, their heart, their being beyond their physical appearance, or in spite of their physical appearance. I'd like to think that maybe we, as human beings, could do so. But to say that what we look like doesn't or shouldn't matter is to deny millions of years of evolution. The fact is, we judge others, and we are judged based on our physical appearance.

Let's return to how we started this chapter, to that huge pimple you had as a teenager. Could you just forget about it? Could you just feel better about it with your will? Could you make others not see it if you behaved like it wasn't there? Unfortunately, no. So, if we know that we judge and are being judged on physical appearance all the time, and it has an impact on how we feel, why not leverage that and make the most of what we have?

There is an undeniable connection between looking good and feeling good. So instead of feeling guilty about working on our appearance, why not embrace it? If we know our appearance so deeply affects how we feel about ourselves and how others feel about us, why deny it? Why should you have one moment of guilt when you consider doing something to alter your appearance for the better? Alternatively, you can view your steps toward plastic surgery or a non-surgical cosmetic procedure as a positive statement to the world. Think of it as a way of displaying and reflecting the health, vitality, beauty, and youth that you feel on the inside to the outside world.

When people make a change, their confidence can soar. They look better, they feel better, and their brain receives positive feedback from others around them. A powerful, positive feedback loop develops, resulting in a massive improvement in self-image and self-confidence. I started the chapter with a quote from a patient of mine who aptly put her finger on the connection between looking good and feeling good. Now let's hear from the same patient again, the holistic practitioner, when asked how surgery has changed her: "When I am tired after a long day and I look in the mirror, that fatigue is not reflected on my face as it was in the past. It does give me an added boost of energy! My inner vitality becomes enlivened!" This is a prime example of the "outer" positively affecting the "inner."

5

Changing Your Appearance through Plastic Surgery Is Not Giving In to Objectification, Sexism, or Extremism

Maybe you're reading this book and it has really pissed you off. In fact, you're so angry, you want to stop reading or throw the book in the trash. Maybe you still completely disagree. "Are you kidding me? A story about some pathetic aging executive who has to get plastic surgery to make her husband pay attention to her? Americans have the right opinion of people who get plastic surgery: it's for the vapid and vain, and it certainly leads to weird-looking people.

You're telling me that to improve my own self-image, I have to alter my physical appearance? That is ridiculous. I don't care what others think of the way I look, even if humans are, as you say, 'intensely visual and social.' I am a more balanced and strong person, and my self-image is completely under my control. Plastic surgery is giving in to objectification and sexism, and it's extreme!"

I am sure, despite some very compelling arguments and illustrations to the contrary, some of you still have these feelings. I am not here to convince anyone who holds dear to these negative opinions about physical transformation through plastic surgery to completely change their views. As I discussed in the introduction, my point in writing this book is not to convert people who just plain feel plastic surgery is not right for them, and believe it never will be. My aim is to provide support for those who are struggling with the decision of whether or not to have plastic surgery. I wrote this book for patients who are conflicted and feel the guilt, worry, or shame that can be associated with pursuing plastic surgery or non-surgical enhancement.

There are a lot of other issues you may be wrestling with and arguments you may be facing within yourself or from others. So, in this chapter, we'll further explore some of these arguments and examine the issues of objectification, sexism, and extremism.

THE ISSUE OF OBJECTIFICATION

The argument that altering your appearance gives in to objectification goes something like this: "I have to care about how I look because other people are judging me and even go to the extent of changing my looks through plastic surgery? This is just giving in to objectification. I am not an object. I am a person and demand to be seen that way." Objectification is a person being perceived as a thing or object first and foremost and being treated as such without consideration for the feelings and emotions of the person.

No one likes to be objectified. Objectification not only hurts emotionally—it allows humans to interact with one another in inhumane ways. Sexual harassment and even assault is a prime example of objectification, and unfortunately, it happens all too often. Listening to the news over a certain period, it seemed a new sexual predator was uncovered in Hollywood or the media almost every day: Bill Cosby (convicted), Harvey Weinstein (convicted), Anthony Weiner (convicted), and Bill O'Reilly (alleged). Their horrific acts were perpetrated on women without consideration for their feelings, well-being, or humanity, because they were viewed as objects to be used to fill deranged sexual needs. And murder, the most inhumane act and greatest sin, is also an act of detachment and objectification. How else could you explain the cruel indifference of murderers and serial killers? John Wayne Gacy, Jeffery Dahmer, and Ted Bundy exhibited the ultimate objectification of others that makes it possible for people to become not only inhuman, but utter monsters.

However, there are some instances where objectification, or a certain degree of detachment in human interaction, is not used for evil, but is actually a necessary tool for doing good. Performing surgery is the first thing that comes to mind. This might sound a little strange because I have wonderful relationships with my patients, and very profound and deep interactions with them before we step in the operating room. However, once we cross that threshold, the person becomes a nose, a face, or an eyelid. They become a collection of parts to be cut, pulled, tucked, reshaped, and stitched to perfection. Objectification allows me to do what I do in the operating room.

As we established, human beings are intensely visual and social. We essentially communicate subliminally, in a blink, with visual and social cues and interpret that data rapidly in our brains. Remember, the brain is a visual judgment machine. But is this complex function of the brain the same thing as objectifying or seeing someone only for what they look like? In most instances, I would say no. The cliché of the ogling construction worker or fifteen-year-old boy who looks at an attractive, unsuspecting woman or girl and thinks just one thing is clearly an example of objectification. These hardly qualify as true human interactions.

Now, imagine that unsuspecting woman stops and speaks

to the construction worker because she hears catcalls or a whistle, and doesn't take kindly to being treated like an object. This is where the true human interaction begins. Imagine her voice is more authoritative than he expected; she speaks with a different tone and cadence, using lawyerly words, and her expression changes to one of consternation and indignation. The construction worker's brain suddenly gets a whole new picture.

He unconsciously takes in the scene: her hair is pulled back in a bun with slight graying at the temples. She has a muscular build and appears to be his physical match, and her eyes, while a beautiful green, have a searing, "I see right through you" quality. Suddenly, he feels like a jerk, like a fourth-grade schoolboy. How did this change of heart happen in thirty seconds? Is it only the words or the tone the woman used that had this tough construction worker shaking in his boots? I say no. Even in this instance, where someone tries to see someone else merely for their looks or as an object, those very same looks are used to send quite a different message. And while what we say and how we say it matters, much more of our communication is visual and subliminal than we realize.

Caring about how you look is not giving in to objectification or inviting people to consider you only on the basis of your appearance. It is capitalizing on a fundamental fact about the way human beings communicate. Instead of feeling like you are giving in or selling out by changing the way you look to make yourself or others happy, why not see it as empowering yourself? You're communicating your inner beauty, inner strength, and inner vitality to the world in a way that most human beings will first and foremost receive that information: visually.

THE ISSUE OF SEXISM

Yet another argument plastic surgery haters may present (are you still there?) is that caring so much about your appearance as to alter it through plastic surgery is clearly driven by a sexist ideology. If you are a potential patient, you may worry you are perpetuating sexism by focusing on your looks to the extent that you'd have surgery to better your appearance. Truth be told, 90 percent of my patients are women. And despite the annual media hype proclaiming the "year of the man" in aesthetic industry magazines, and even boutique practices springing up that cater exclusively to men, those statistics barely budge.

There does seem to be a double standard when it comes to appearance. A male with some graying in his beard appears "distinguished," but a woman with some graying in her temples is "old." Aging men can still be viewed as attractive, even as sex symbols. A case in point: George Clooney was named sexiest man alive in 2006 at the age of forty-five. When have you ever seen a woman over the age of thirty on the cover of *Sports Illustrated*? Or how about the small number of female reporters, sportscasters, and actresses who are able to continue their careers well into their sixth and seventh decades versus the number of men. Granted, there are plenty of exceptions where women have had successful careers in the media and Hollywood past their "prime." For example, celebrities like Barbara Walters, Jane Fonda, Greta Van Susteren, Kris Jenner, Celine Dion, Madonna, Kathy Lee Gifford, Cher, and Jennifer Lopez have been very successful in the spotlight later in life and, perhaps not coincidentally, they've all had plastic surgery or non-surgical cosmetic procedures. Undoubtedly, there is plenty of sexism and ageism in the media and in the world of entertainment.

However, the reasons women turn toward plastic surgery in higher numbers than men are more complex than sexism alone. The fact is, women of all ages just seem to care more about their appearance, regardless of what the men around them think. Women preen, paint, poke, and prod their faces and bodies into colors, shapes, and sizes they find more attractive. This seems to go well beyond the biological drive to attract a mate. I have female patients in their eighties who have been married for sixty years, and their husbands don't give a damn what they look like. Likewise, these female octogenarians could care less about what their husbands think of their appearance. "I am doing this for myself!" they say. And I believe them.

The drive for women to appear beautiful to the world comes from a much deeper place. It is rooted in biology and evolution. We talked about how human beings communicate visually, and that a huge amount of social information is gathered from the face and appearance. While men are often credited with being more "visual," the truth is 65 percent of the entire population, male and female, are visual learners.[16]

Women are certainly more social. They form deeper bonds and connections and are more in tune to feedback from others, including feedback on appearance. In other words, women have a more powerful visual/social sense. How else do you explain the forty-year-old guy with the beer gut peering into the mirror in his bathing suit and exclaiming: "I look pretty good, don't I?" In case you're wondering, this is not an individual, autobiographical statement. Men are clueless when it comes to appearance. They don't care about the way they look as much, because they don't pick up on or thrive on the feedback they get from others about the way they look.

Besides social oblivion, there are other reasons why men don't seek out plastic surgery or non-surgical treatments as often as women. Men, on average, show signs of facial aging more slowly than women. Men have thicker, more sebaceous skin with abundant hair follicles. One of the major

---

16   Heather A. Rupp and Kim Wallen, "Sex Differences in Response to Visual Sexual Stimuli: A Review," Archives of Sexual Behavior, 37, no. 2 (2008): 206–18.

factors in facial aging is a literal thinning of the facial skin. The three key components of skin are: collagen, which gives skin its structure; elastin, which gives skin its snap; and hyaluronic acid, which gives skin its hydration and plumpness. Our skin loses 1 percent of collagen every year after the age of twenty. Hyaluronic acid and elastin undergo similar declines, albeit at different rates. If you start out with thicker skin as men do, you have a major advantage, as this loss of key skin components will take a longer time to wreak havoc and to ultimately show wrinkles. This advantage also goes for other parts of the face that undergo aging, particularly the underlying facial bones and muscles. These are generally bigger and thicker in men to start, so they atrophy or shrink less with age.

So, while those who argue that women are driven to pursue plastic surgery due to a sexist double standard may be right, it's not the whole story. In fact, it may be a very small part of the story. The bigger picture is rooted in some key biological and sociological differences between the sexes. Women show signs of aging a bit faster because of thinner skin and other facets of the facial aging process. And, as we established, women have a keener visual/social sense than men. They are more attuned to what others look like and how they appear to others. It's more important to them to look good not only to please men, but to please each other, and most importantly, to please themselves. Ironically, in this sense, embracing the idea of maximizing your appearance through non-surgical treatments or plastic surgery may be viewed as more female or even, dare I say, "feminist."

If you are facing pressure or shaming from others who say caring about your appearance or undergoing plastic surgery is giving in to sexism, you may now counter their argument with biological and sociological facts. You are simply maximizing your appearance to your social advantage and embracing who and what you are: a female. I would argue that the pursuit of looking your best at any age may be a more feminist, empowering, and life-affirming approach than allowing "nature to take its course." It falls on the sword of the feminist double standard.

IS PLASTIC SURGERY "EXTREME"?

Maybe you're not worried about these other big societal issues like being accused of giving in to objectification or sexism, but you and others around you are more concerned about you doing something "extreme." After all, isn't caring so much about how you look to the extent that you would alter yourself with a medical procedure clearly a sign of taking things to the extreme?

Think about the number of things we do to our bodies on a daily basis to maintain our social standing. We wash our bodies, cut our nails, primp our hair, brush our teeth, and the list goes on and on. Why do we do any amount of grooming? Yes, we do like smelling clean, and it does feel good to be well groomed, but isn't it largely to fit in with our social peers and attract others? Or, at the very least, to keep them from running away? Now, imagine if you were to stop grooming, even for a few days. Cut out showering, trimming your nails, cutting your hair, or doing your makeup for a while, and see if it impacts how others react to you.

You don't really have to use your imagination to see how others might react to your lack of grooming. For example, if you've spent any time in a city, you know how people react to the homeless. No matter how saintly we may hope to be, the gut, human reaction to one who is ungroomed is one of aversion and avoidance. Why? Our brain processes those visual and social cues like the long hair, unkempt beard, bad smell, and long nails as signs that the person could be potentially dangerous to our well-being or, at the very least, unpleasant to be around. This initiates our fight-or-flight response. Although we are capable of calling on our higher nature and offering compassion and help, our initial reaction is usually one of repulsion. We must overcome this reaction if we are to offer a helping hand.

Now, let's talk about things that affect our appearance beyond the scope of basic grooming. How about a big, hairy mole on our chin, bad acne, or big, scaly brown patches on our face? How do these lesions affect our social interactions? My elementary-school librarian, God rest her soul, was a very kind and loving teacher. She also had a huge, scary mole on her chin, sprouting hair from its center. One of the things kids loved about her was that she gave us Cheerios for answering questions correctly. (Hey, it was the seventies, and we were happy with much less). Despite her kindness, kids whispered, stared at her chin, and avoided hugs or contact because of her scary mole. After all, witches had moles, not teachers. I ponder how many interactions with students and other teachers or administrators were altered for her because of this physical flaw. Looking back, I wonder why she never cared to have this elephant in the room removed. Maybe she tried and could not find the right doctor to do it. Would removing this mole have been considered altering her appearance, or basic grooming? Would it be considered an extreme measure to undergo a medical procedure to have this mole removed? Most people would probably say no, and might even consider the procedure to be necessary.

Now let's think about subtler physical flaws: the dark circles under the eyes, crow's feet, the jowls, or other signs of aging. What signals do these kinds of physical flaws send out? Tiredness, exhaustion, even perhaps illness. Patients frequently come into my office because of the off-handed comment from their friends or colleagues: "Did you get enough sleep last night?" If you hear that a few times a week from more than one person, pretty soon you get the hint. So, the patient comes to my office to have this situation remedied. He or she has the surgical procedure, and the tired look is gone. They look exactly like themselves, except the physical flaw that was drawing so much attention is gone.

Do you think this patient crossed the line into being radical or extreme? Where exactly is the line where intervention to change the way we look and appear to others becomes extreme? The line is not so clear. People have plastic surgery for some of the very same reasons we wash our hair, cut our nails, and generally take care of the way we present ourselves. Although plastic surgery is a bit more involved than combing our hair, no one takes issue with or judges someone for combing their hair. No one gets shamed because they regularly take showers, but the plastic surgery patient must frequently hide, lie, conceal, and cover what they've done for fear of social retribution from friends or family.

People who have an axe to grind with plastic surgery are missing the point, whether they are acting out of their own fears, preconceived notions, misinformation, or ignorance. Most people don't undergo these medical procedures because they are vain, conceited, self-centered, insecure, or prone to extreme measures. Most people who have plastic surgery are grounded, healthy people who have something they simply want to improve about their appearance. Instead of denying that others will judge them, good or bad, for what they present to the world, plastic surgery patients accept this reality. They take a more pragmatic approach to dealing with their physical insecurities, and they get rid of them.

By having the guts to do something about their physical flaws, they are making the best of the image they present to the world, and they improve their image of themselves. The beautiful thing to witness, as I have many times, is that these positive transformations can be just as much mental or spiritual as they are physical. As shocking as it may sound, having plastic surgery, in this sense, can be as healthy mentally and physically as taking care of yourself through any other means such as exercise, diet, healthy habits, or meditation.

6

The Attractiveness Advantage: Why It's Smart to Care about How You Look

In the last chapter, we talked about various objections people have to plastic surgery and non-surgical procedures: some view it as objectification, or as sexist or extreme. We considered the alternative perspective and saw that on the contrary, these procedures can be empowering, feminist (if you happen to be female), pragmatic, and even mentally and physically healthy. Now, what if I told you maximizing your appearance through medical enhancement or rejuvenation not only is pragmatic, but may offer you a distinct advantage in life?

Of course, variables other than attractiveness factor into the equation for success, but when all things are equal (or even unequal), the person with the better smile, stronger chin, more delicate nose, brighter eyes, or even taller height gets the nod. This is the essence of the "attractiveness advantage."

THE ATTRACTIVENESS ADVANTAGE

While it may seem wrong that we, as human beings, could be so biased by such a trivial thing as someone's appearance, we cannot argue with the biological facts. The attractiveness advantage is not learned, but appears to be hardwired into our brains. Even babies judge faces according to their beauty and show a clear, discernible preference toward gazing at attractive faces.[17] Are these babies being superficial and overly focused on vanity? No, they are being biologically practical. Their brains are hardwired to fix their gaze on attractive people who seem most healthy, most vital, and most capable of offering what babies need most: help fulfilling their own biological needs for safety, shelter, and food.

Of course, the attractiveness advantage continues to impact how we think well past childhood. The human brain recognizes patterns, and this is what scientists call the "heuristic" nature of the brain—the propensity of the brain to take shortcuts, develop rules, and ascribe meaning (i.e., "When I see 'x', it means 'y'"). Our brains do this naturally with

17   https://www.newscientist.com/article/
      dn6355-babies-prefer-to-gaze-upon-beautiful-faces/

almost everything we hear, see, feel, and taste. The brain is, of course, heuristic when it comes to how we see other people as well. Our brains will make judgments about other people based on their physical attributes, even down to individual facial features and body parts.

How might this work? Let's do an exercise using the chin as an example. In both males and females, there is an ideal chin shape and size in proportion to the rest of the face. One of the ways we analyze chins in facial plastic surgery is by the concept of equal thirds. At the front view, the face should have equal thirds roughly from the hairline to the eyes, from the eyes to the base of the nose, and from mid-lip to the chin.

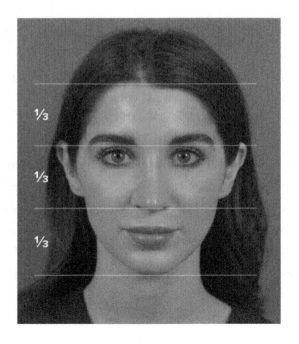

People with small chins are "deficient" in the lower third. At the side view, the chin should stick out or project from the face and meet a line dropped from the pink part of the lower lip. When the chin doesn't do this, in plastic surgery we say that the chin does not have "adequate projection." This is how facial plastic surgeons, as doctors, interpret the visual data: very objectively and without emotional judgment.

However, this is not how we, as human beings, view the same face. The hardwired programs of the brain tell us something very different on a social/emotional level about this facial attribute. Think about a man with a small, mousy chin, big nose, and maybe a big Adam's apple. We take the visual image and immediately ascribe the visual characteristics of the person to their personality and consider them to be mousy, timid, shy, and maybe even a bit simple. Think about how this is reinforced by our culture. I'm sure you can recall one or two cartoons from childhood that depicted this exact visual image and social interpretation.

Now let's consider the opposite: a chin that projects strongly, and a defined jawline that's maybe even a little cleft. How do we visually interpret that? That male is viewed as strong, virile, and maybe even superhuman, like Superman. But if the chin, on the other hand, is too big or exaggerated, maybe like Jay Leno's or Inspector Gadget's, it's interpreted as comical or clown-like.

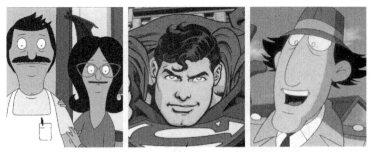

Left: Alamy stock photo/AF archive. Center: Alamy stock photo/Contributor Cum Okolo. Right: Alamy stock photo/Contributor Moviestore Collection Ltd.

Let's consider another body part for this exercise: the nose. Nasal interpretation and nasal surgery are considered one of the most complex exercises and operations in all of plastic surgery. There are more rules dictating the aesthetic ideal with the nose than any other body part, and I will mention some of them here. The nose should have a smooth, straight bridge without bumps or irregularities. The nose should be roughly a 3:4:5 triangle.

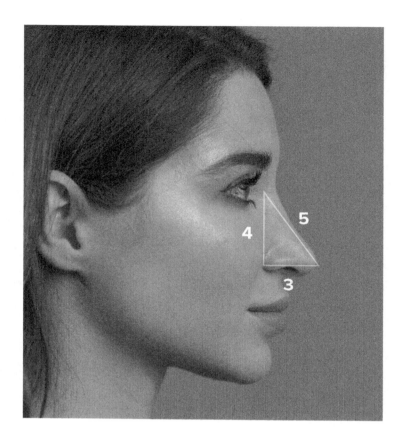

The nasal tip should project or stick out from the plane of the face (where it begins between the eyes) to about the length of the upper lip. And there are many, many more rules.

As facial plastic surgeons, our minds judge what we see scientifically and objectively, and we determine the best surgical plan to modify the nose to reach the ideal aesthetic outcome. However, we are *trained* to think that way. On a more basic level, our brains judge people's faces (and noses for that matter) heuristically. Our brain uses shortcuts, sub-consciously and emotionally.

Think about a big nose with a large bump and downward hook to the nasal tip.

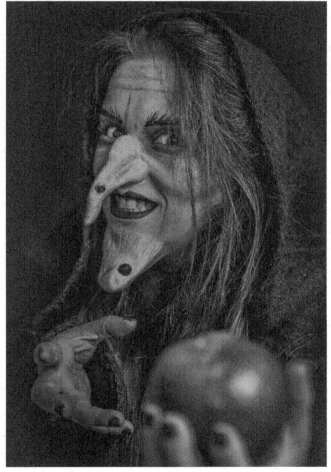

Alamy photographer: Jose Antonio Garcia Sosa

What kind of character traits do we usually ascribe to a person with this physical feature? Unlikeable, cunning, maybe even evil. After all, this is the kind of nose drawn on witches. Contrastingly, a nose with a straight/narrow bridge and tip to match with either a slight incline (for women) or ninety-degree tip angle (for men) is considered delicate, demure, and refined.

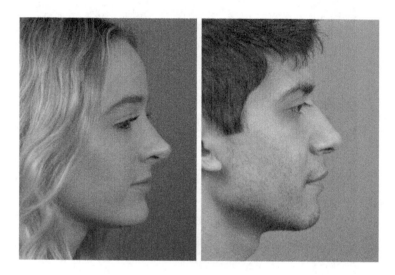

This is the nose of a prince or princess.

You can take almost any physical feature, repeat the same exercise, and easily see how our brains ascribe meaning to bodily features based on their shape, size, and configuration. Assessing other people's attractiveness is hardwired into our brains from birth, and our brain takes shortcuts when it comes to judging people based on their physical characteristics. Judging and being judged by others based on looks is not a sin, vanity, or a tendency toward the trivial. Rather, it is a biological function of the human brain.

The attractiveness advantage plays a part in almost every sphere of human interaction. Clearly, physical attractiveness is one of the most important factors for men and women (although they don't like to admit it) in courtship and mating. When meeting someone of the opposite or same sex, depending on your orientation, your brain does a rapid-fire analysis of their physical appearance. Do they have nice eyes, good cheekbones, a nice chin, nose, chest, butt, hips, legs, etc.? In fact, that might be all you can focus on when you first meet a potential mate. Why does the brain put in so much time and energy and pump us full of exciting chemicals like endorphins to make this initial attraction phase so exciting, memorable, and even all-consuming? Because selecting a mate is one of the most important biological choices we will make!

Even as the evolved and prescient beings we are, we're just like every other organism on this planet. We're no different than viruses in that we have a strong biological drive to pass on our genes. If we didn't, human beings would not be successful as a species. Since we have little or no ability to "see" someone's genes, we do it the old-fashioned way by interpreting physical traits as an outward expression of inner health, vitality, and biological worthiness as a mate.

For example, why are men so attracted to the hips, pelvis, and butt area? Have you ever heard the expression "child-bearing hips"? Men, in focusing on the hips, are assessing a woman's ability to successfully have offspring. In the past, women with narrower hips and a flatter butt were more likely to die during childbirth when we didn't have access to C-sections. And if the females died during childbirth, the male's genes would not be passed on.

Why are women so attracted to men with muscular chests, arms, shoulders? It's because someone with this physical prowess was more able to protect her family unit from would-be assailants, of which there were many during our evolution. If the family unit was attacked or killed, her genes would not be passed on.

OTHER IMPLICATIONS OF THE ATTRACTIVENESS ADVANTAGE

Now that we have taken all the fun out of falling in love, let's talk about other areas of life where the attractiveness advantage comes into play. Clearly, being attractive gives a distinct advantage when seeking employment for a whole host of careers. Really, every career. Hollywood is the most obvious example. Our leading men and women are typically the epitome of physical prowess and attractiveness. George Clooney, Carey Grant, Paul Newman, and Brad Pitt are just some examples of attractiveness being a prerequisite for a leading man. And for women, Grace Kelly, Audrey Hepburn, Angelina Jolie, and Julia Roberts come to mind as leading ladies in the beauty department.

If you are less than perfect, you become more of a character actor (e.g., Al Pacino or Meryl Streep). In these roles, you have to bring more personality to the table. Brooding, staring off into the distance, or striking a seductive pose is simply not enough. These actors need to connect with us in other ways. If you are less attractive, short, or overweight (e.g., Adam Sandler, Danny Devito, or Melissa McCarthy), you have to work even harder to make the audience like you. You have to bring even *more* personality into the equation and make us laugh to make it on the big screen.

Outside of Hollywood, in almost every form of visual media, there is an advantage to being attractive. Even in the news, which can be very serious business, looks matter. Why does Fox News have a lot of attractive, blond, female news personalities? It's because they very astutely know how to attract their audience, mostly middle-aged white males. While it's obvious that it is important to be attractive in Hollywood and on TV, as careers sometimes rise and fall with levels of attractiveness, it may be less obvious in other spheres.

How about in politics and business? Consider a simple physical trait: height. Height conveys command, physical strength, and prowess, which are important qualities for a commander in chief and captains of industry. Of the forty-five American Presidents, thirty-nine of them have been above the height of the average American male, which is about 5'8". In business, chief executive officers, who represent the business equivalent of "commanders in chief," are almost universally taller with 90 percent of Fortune 500 CEOs being above average height (e.g., Tim Cook of Apple, Sir Richard Branson of Virgin Group, and Elon Musk of Tesla). Multiple studies have also shown that for every inch of height above average, you earn an additional 1.8 percent in annual wages.[18] But our predilection for picking more attractive people to lead us goes way beyond height.

In presidential politics, despite all the speeches, discussion of the issues, and plans for the future, we usually choose the more likable (i.e., attractive) candidate. The "who would you rather have a beer with?" contest is one of the litmus tests used by political pundits. It essentially gauges who is more relatable to a wider array of people. Think about the races between JFK and Nixon, Clinton and Dole, George H. W. Bush and Dukakis, and Obama and McCain. In almost every race, the more attractive candidate got the nod. If you are old enough to remember or have seen an image of the jowly older Richard Nixon sweating profusely in a debate against the cool, suave Kennedy, you have seen a crystal-clear example of the attractiveness advantage in politics.

---

18   Joe Pinsker, ""The Financial Perks of Being Tall: An Extra Inch Correlates with an Estimated $800 in Increased Annual Earnings," *The Atlantic*, May 18, 2015.

Attractive presidents are more likely to be widely popular, like JFK, Ronald Reagan, or Bill Clinton, and are more likely to get a pass on missteps while in office.

Outside of Hollywood, the media, and politics, it's hard to imagine that physical appearance and the attractiveness advantage does not factor into the equation in interviewing, hiring, and climbing to the top of almost any occupation. Intuitively, we all know this. When we go for a job interview, we spend as much time preparing our look as we do our résumé. We may get a haircut, a new suit, our nails done, and a clean shave. We certainly do everything to look our best and use the attractiveness advantage *to our advantage* when seeking a job.

The *Small Business Chronicle* says: "Once hired, better-looking people earn more on average. According to 'Forbes' magazine, attractiveness brings a 5 percent boost in earnings. Taller-than-average males receive a 6 percent premium over their average peers. A woman 5-feet-7 also earns $5,250 more per year than one 5 inches shorter. However, negative physical traits diminish earning power. Shorter-than-average men receive 4 percent less in salary than those with average height, and obese women suffer a 5 percent loss in wages. General unattractiveness brings a wage loss in the range of 7 to 9 percent."[19]

---

19   https://smallbusiness.chron.com/attractive-people-advantage-workplace-15421.html

Even CEOs, who are at the very pinnacle of a business, are not immune to being judged based on their looks. CEOs are most often elected by a company board for their business acumen, leadership skills, and well, their attractiveness. And once in office, their attractiveness continues to play a role in their perceived success. From the *Chief Executive:* "Researchers examined whether and how the appearance of CEOs affects shareholder value. They came up with a 'Facial Attractiveness Index' of 677 CEOs from the S&P 500 companies based on their facial geometry. CEOs with a higher Facial Attractiveness Index were found to be associated with better stock returns around their first days on the job, and higher acquirer returns upon acquisition announcements."[20]

Some CEOs and business titans, like Jeff Bezos, Mark Zuckerberg, and Elon Musk, are not exactly known for their devilish good looks, but these guys started their own companies. However, even these business geniuses don't get a pass; their success comes with a lot of effort in grooming and making themselves appear as attractive as possible to lead their teams.

In sum, attractiveness provides a clear advantage in almost every sphere of human interaction and endeavor, from courtship to career. Knowing this fact, why should anyone who endeavors to become more attractive through plastic surgery be made to feel guilty, dumb, or superficial?

20 https://chiefexecutive.net/does-the-ceo-have-to-be-attractive-to-succeed/

Isn't maximizing your attractiveness advantage through any means possible really the smart play here? By making yourself appear as attractive as possible, you maximize your chances of success and endeavor to make the most out of your life, which clearly isn't dumb, superficial, or a reason to feel guilt.

THE EFFECTS OF AGING ON THE ATTRACTIVENESS ADVANTAGE

Allow me to state some bad news that may already be blatantly obvious to you: the attractiveness advantage declines with age. This may, in fact, be the very reason you decided to read this book. While all of us are reminded every day when we look in the mirror that our looks are waning, we may not think about the impact this can have on our lives, or how our attractiveness advantage is slipping away.

Ageism in the workplace is a well-known phenomenon, and study after study shows how an employer's impression of a potential candidate or an employee's productivity is biased by their age and appearance. People who appear older are at a distinct disadvantage in the workplace. Yes, there are certain instances where appearing a bit older and wiser may, in fact, land you the job because you are perceived as more experienced or seasoned, but on average, the older or more aged you appear, the less likely you are to land a job, excel, or even keep your current job.

A study by the company Hiscox in 2019 on ageism in the workplace, which surveyed people over the age of forty, found that more than 36 percent of workers felt their age prevented them from getting a job, 21 percent of workers felt they had been discriminated against because of their age, and 26 percent felt there was some risk they could lose their current job because of their age. There is no denying that your apparent age affects how you are perceived by your superiors and coworkers. For example, one study found that assertiveness in the workplace, while a positive trait in youth, is interpreted more negatively when the person is older.[21]

Why does one's apparent age affect how they are perceived by others? Earlier in the chapter, we discussed the "heuristic" nature of the human brain. To refresh your memory, that is the linking of certain physical or visual cues with preconceived notions. Not surprisingly, our brains function the same way when they are looking at traits of the aging human face.

HOW OUR FACE CAN BELIE OUR EMOTIONS BUT REFLECT OUR HEALTH

Let's look at some common aging problems and see what meaning these images conjure up. Take a look at image 10.

---

21   M. North and S. Fiske, "Act Your (Old) Age: Prescriptive, Ageist Biases over Succession, Identity, and Consumption," *Personality and Social Psychology Bulletin* 39, 6 (2013): 720–34.

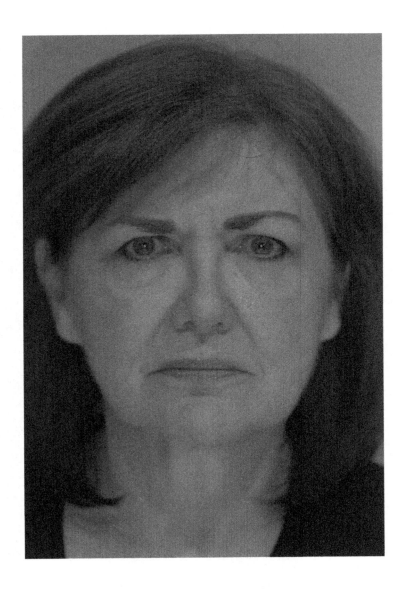

What do you think of this person? They look angry, don't they? The brows have fallen down and inward. The "frown lines" or "elevens" have deepened. Why does the brain interpret this image as someone being angry? Because we make this very same expression when we are angry.

In anger, our corrugator and procerus muscles draw the eyebrows downward and inward, causing furrowing, as seen in image 11.

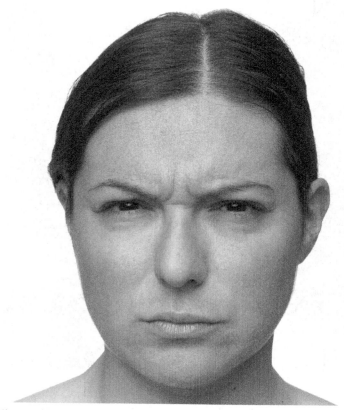

Shutterstock: ZoneCreative

In the aging brow, the angry expression never entirely goes away because the brows are chronically drawn downward and inward, not only by tonic muscle contraction, but also by drooping of the tissues due to gravity. When the muscles of the aging brow are chemically or surgically relaxed, however, the angry expression goes away. See image 12, of the same patient in image 10, following surgical (endoscopic) browlift:

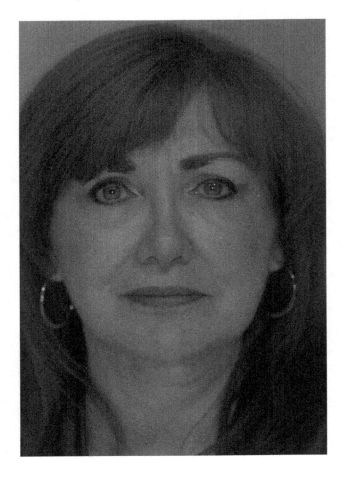

Take a look at image 13.

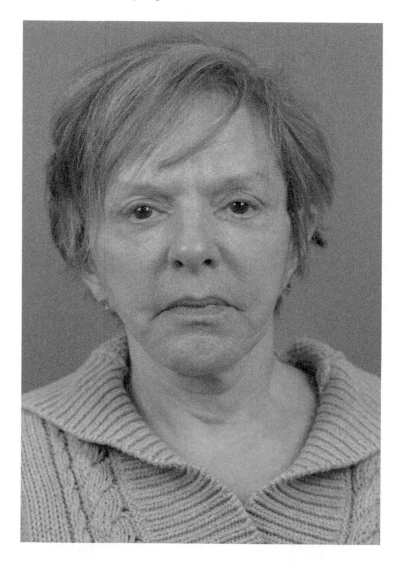

What do you think of this person? They seem sad, down, and/or depressed, don't they? The sagging lower face, in particular, and the droopy corners of the mouth give this impression. Why? It's because when we are sad or depressed, we activate the muscles that cause the corners of the mouth to sag, as we can see in image 14.

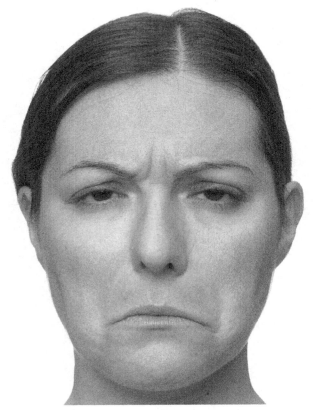

Shutterstock: ZoneCreative

In the aging face, unfortunately, this expression can become permanent due to gravity and tonic muscle contraction. But when the corners of the mouth are no longer downturned, the sad expression goes away. Image 15 shows the same patient from image 13, following a corner of the mouth lift.

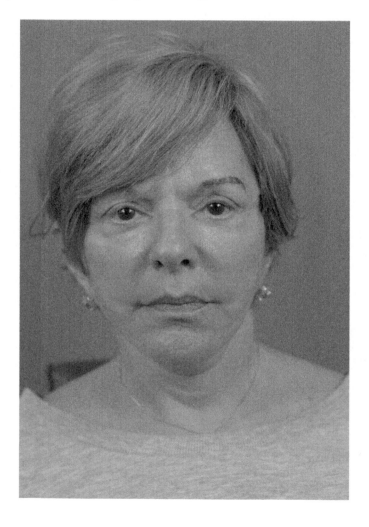

How about this image?

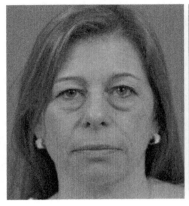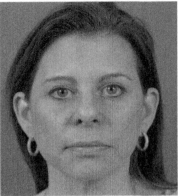

We already discussed this one in earlier chapters. The photo on the left shows how dark circles or eye bags give the impression that someone is tired, exhausted, or even ill. Why? Because many illnesses cause fatigue and dark circles or bags under the eyes. In the aging face, due to volume-related changes around the eyes, this tired look can be permanent. The photo on the right depicts how this looks when corrected with a lower blepharoplasty (removal or repositioning of the lower eyelid bags) and microfat transfer to take fat from one part of the body via liposuction and inject it into the face.

How about when we see the old turkey neck? We may think that person is well past their prime, overweight, or unhealthy. When the turkey neck is gone, the person appears healthier, as seen in image 17:

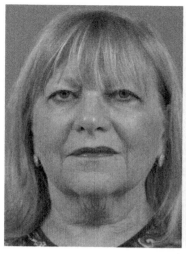 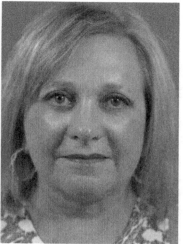

These issues are not just theoretical. These are some of the most common complaints I hear from patients every day. "Doc, everyone keeps telling me I look angry, and I tell them I am perfectly happy. It's so frustrating!" "People are telling me I look sad and down. I hate how the corners of my mouth droop down, and how my neck has a turkey waddle." And the patient with eye bags says, "If I have to hear one more time: 'You look tired, did you get enough sleep?' I'll scream!"

Eye bags and turkey waddles are probably two of the most common problems, and patients will frequently say they feel healthy, young, and vital, but others don't see them that way. They are tired of being asked if they feel okay or if they are tired. In our discussions, the exasperation patients feel when they repeatedly hear these comments is palpable. "I feel great, but people keep telling me I look tired or sick. There is absolutely nothing wrong with me!" You might agree they are right to be angry. After all, just because someone looks older or has eye bags doesn't mean they are unhealthy. Common sense says that is ridiculous. It is just the way we look on the outside; our appearance has nothing to do with our actual health. Why do our brains make these assumptions?

Our brains, in making these connections, may be smarter than we think. The surprising fact is, there is a strong correlation between physical appearance and internal (physiologic) health. Making this judgment is a part of basic medical training. In medical training, we are taught to record whether someone "looks their stated age" or "looks older than their stated age." In actuality, physicians are pretty good at judging someone's health by the way they look.

Research has shown a strong correlation between individuals who appeared greater than or equal to ten years their stated age and poor health. A 2012 study presented at the American Heart Association scientific session found that those who had three to four signs of aging—receding hairline at the temples, baldness at the head's crown, earlobe crease, or yellow fatty deposits around the eyelid (xanthelasma)— had a 57 percent increased risk for heart attack, and a 39 percent increased risk for heart disease. "The visible signs of aging reflect physiologic or biological age, not chronological age, and are independent of chronological age," said Anne Tybjaerg-Hansen, MD, the study's senior author and Professor of Clinical Biochemistry at the University of Copenhagen in Denmark.[22] So, looking old is a clear and accurate sign to others that you are, in fact, less healthy, less vital, and perhaps less capable.

Now, of course, having plastic surgery won't automatically make you healthier on the inside. It will just make you *appear* healthier. While no data currently exists, I wouldn't be surprised if over time patients who have had plastic surgery become healthier as a result of restored confidence, increased happiness, and their efforts to optimize and maintain their results with healthy choices.

In this chapter, we learned that the attractiveness advantage is a pervasive fact of life. We are born with a predilection toward attractive faces, and the attractiveness advantage is hardwired into our brains. Given the brain's heuristic programming, we can't help but associate certain physical traits with particular attributes, both positive and negative. The attractiveness advantage plays a role in almost every sphere of life: our choices of mates, the media, politics, and the workplace. The attractiveness advantage declines as we age, as evidenced by ageism in the workplace. Our brains make heuristic judgments when it comes to the aging face. And you learned that, surprisingly, our external appearance may accurately reflect our internal health and vitality.

22   https://www.sciencedaily.com/releases/2012/11/121106114221.htm

So, to bring us back to the central mantra of this book: "don't feel bad about looking good." If you are seeking to improve your appearance at any age, whether through diet, exercise, non-surgical intervention, or plastic surgery, you are making a smart play. There is nothing wrong with wanting your outward appearance to reflect your inner health, vitality, and zest for life. You are maximizing your attractiveness advantage, which can have profound effects in every aspect of your life.

7

The Guilt over Defying Nature: Why Aging "Gracefully" Doesn't Always Mean "Naturally"

So, maybe you're thinking to yourself, "I know I don't look as good as I used to, but I just have to accept it and age gracefully." You may harbor guilt, as many do, about trying to look younger with plastic surgery or non-surgical anti-aging procedures. You may be shamed or even mocked by others for even contemplating it.

You're not alone. A lot of people have worry and guilt when they consider aesthetic medicine or plastic surgery because they get a nagging feeling that maybe it isn't right to fool with Mother Nature. I've even heard people say they know they will be punished, or that something is bound to go wrong with their procedure because they are "being so vain." This anxiety and guilt is reinforced every few years by the aging celebrity who has an aha moment and swears off plastic surgery. "I am not going to cut myself anymore. I can pretend I'm not vain," declared Jane Fonda at eighty-two, after spending most of her life having procedures. Sharon Osborne also had this epiphany in 2012 and "swore off" plastic surgery, only to reverse course and undergo a major facelift in 2019. These declarations only serve to reinforce the stereotypical notion that plastic surgery and aesthetic medicine are somehow morally wrong. Anyone who considers them has an addiction that must be broken, because it is "unnatural."

But what exactly is "natural" when it comes to aging? Is "letting nature do its thing" and embracing the extra pounds, dark circles under the eyes, and degradation of your face and body somehow graceful? In the last chapter, we discussed the attractiveness advantage and the harsh reality of its decline with age. We touched on ageism in society and in the workplace. We discussed how facial aging can send the wrong visual cues or signals to the brain, causing people to discount, dismiss, or overlook you. They may consider you irrelevant, less than capable, or past your prime.

In this chapter, we will explore what aging is both at the microscopic (invisible) and macroscopic (visible) levels. We will learn how the degradation of our tissues leads to our aged appearance. Armed with this understanding of the aging process, we can shift our perspective of aging from something that should be accepted as "natural" to a malfunction of tissues that can be treated with plastic surgery, just as any other physiologic malfunction is treated with other forms of medicine.

THE BASIC SCIENCE BEHIND AGING

Why does aging happen? Well, it's obvious, right? Time passes, and we get old. More specifically, though, why do our faces, bodies, and minds change at all with the passage of time? In order to understand this, we have to go back to biology class. Cue the time machine: the answer is in our DNA.

DNA stands for deoxyribonucleic acid. Its structure essentially looks like a twisted ladder (the double helix), where its center is made up of pairs of bases, and the sides or rungs are made up of a long sugar strand. It is twisted in and around itself multiple times in a large conglomerate to form a *chromosome*. The chromosomes are located in the cell nucleus. We have twenty-three pairs of chromosomes, including one sex chromosome pair that determines our gender.

What does this have to do with aging? Aging of our outer appearance is really the aging of our cells, or what is called cell *senescence*. Cell senescence is caused, among other things, by the aging of our DNA. Over our lifetimes, our DNA is read and reread by our cells to make the various proteins we need to function. Proteins perform a ton of cell functions, like cell replication and cell signaling. As old cells die, our DNA also is replicated many times over the course of our lifetimes to make new cells. All this protein making and replicating over time takes a toll on our DNA. What was once a clean copy of DNA becomes altered with time.

DNA even has a physical clock called a *telomere*. As the DNA ages, the telomere gets shorter and shorter with time, counting down the life of the cell. The cells basically reflect what happens to us: they produce less energy, can't repair themselves as well, and accordingly, make more mistakes. Almost every human illness that results from aging is due to the aging of our cells.

So, now that we've discussed aging on a basic, cellular level, what happens on a larger (macroscopic) scale? When it comes to aging, the one thing you can count on is constant change. Most would agree that our peak of vitality, strength, and beauty is in our early twenties. Aging changes in the face and body, although subtle, are noticeable for most people by their late twenties to early thirties. Gradual, insidious changes happen between our thirties and age fifty, where a few wrinkles and pounds get added year by year. "Accelerated aging" usually begins after the age of fifty for most people, where the changes seem to accumulate more rapidly and become more blatantly noticeable. Changes in our appearance that reflect our internal decline continue until the point of death. What a cheerful thought! So, what exactly is it about aging that contributes to the way we look as we get older? Is it our skin? Our fat? Our muscles? Our bones? Our organs? The answer is all of the above.

Age-related changes in all of these structures play a part in the way we look as we get older. The changes in the skin have the most profound impacts on our appearance. You learned some of this information earlier when I discussed men's thicker skin and the protection it provides against an aged appearance, but I think it bears repeating. Remember, the skin's collagen content and thickness decline over time, leading to wrinkles. After the age of twenty, collagen production in the skin declines by 1 percent per year. The most important layer for generating new skin cells, the basal cell layer, becomes smaller.

As we also discussed in the chapter about cell aging, the skin cells themselves accumulate more genetic damage. This is why abnormal skin growths seem to multiply as we age. The skin's elastin, the small rubber-band-like proteins in the skin, become disorganized and fragmented. Damage to this protein causes loss of the skin's "elasticity," so our skin hangs and doesn't snap back as we age. The skin doesn't produce as much hyaluronic acid, which is an important substance that attracts water to keep the skin hydrated. As we age, hyaluronic acid decreases in the epidermis, or outer layer of the skin, which essentially decreases its critical function of keeping the water in our skin.

Overall, almost every important component of skin structure and function declines as the skin ages. But, as we discussed, aging is not just "skin deep." Just underneath the skin, over most of the entire body, is a layer of fat. A healthy fat layer gives structural support and plumpness to our facial skin. It is essentially the "stuffing" that makes us look youthful.

NEW DISCOVERIES IN PLASTIC SURGERY

One of the most profound realizations in cosmetic plastic surgery over the past twenty-five years or so is the great impact of volume loss in the aging of the face and body. Prior to this discovery, most surgeons viewed the face and body through a different lens. Gravity was thought to be the main culprit with aging. The entire field of cosmetic surgery revolved around lifting, pulling, and tightening these sagging structures against the pull of gravity. While the effect of gravity and sagging is not to be denied, in most cases, addressing this part of facial and body aging leads to overly pulled, tightened, still wrinkled, and less-than- youthful-looking faces and bodies.

In the early nineties a renewed focus on the effects of volume loss led to a revolution in the field of cosmetic surgery. It was increasingly recognized that aging was due not only to gravity, but also to changes in the volume of skin, fat, and bone. Age-related volume loss occurs in the face beginning in the mid-twenties and progresses throughout life. Take a moment to compare two extremes in age. A baby's face is round, cherubic, and fat, or pleasingly plump. Now, think of the opposite side of the spectrum: an octogenarian. Generally, as people reach their eighties and onward, they begin to exhibit extreme facial wasting with sunken cheeks, temples, and receded upper teeth and jaws. We begin life as nice, plump grapes and eventually become thin, shriveled raisins.

We hit our peaks in our physical appearance in our early twenties, and by our late twenties, we look just a little bit different. Patients in my office note these subtle changes in the way they look, and I can almost always trace it to facial volume loss, the very first thing that happens in facial aging. Aging begins subtly with a little loss of facial fat and bone structure. This progresses slowly and insidiously throughout our lifetimes as we lose volume due to deterioration and changes in fat and bone.

In our thirties through our mid-forties, volume loss is still the main culprit with aging. Gravity and substantial sagging of structures doesn't play much of a role in aging until the mid- to late forties. As aging progresses beyond the mid-forties, only then does it look like skin is really sagging, as aging of the skin and the effects of gravity begin to show. Beyond the age of fifty, volume loss and gravity have more of an equivalent role.

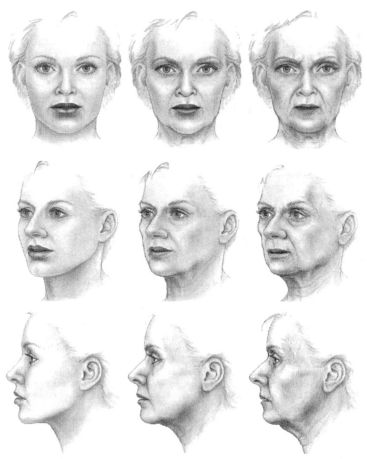

Sydney R. Coleman and Rajiv Grover, "The Anatomy of the Aging Face: Volume Loss and Changes in 3-Dimensional Topography," *Aesthetic Surgery Journal* 26, no. 1 (January 2006): S4–S9.

Let me quote Alanis Morissette here. "Isn't it ironic" that as we age, we lose the fat where we want it (in our faces) and get the fat where we don't need it (in our bellies, hips, and thighs)? As we age, abdominal fat increases due to a decrease in our resting metabolic rate (RMR). Fat is an extremely important structural component of our face. We have eight defined facial fat pads, separated by facial ligaments or connective tissue. The fat pad under our eyes, for example, is called the *sub-orbicularis oculi fat pad* or "Soof" for short. One of the main fat pads in our cheeks is called the *malar fat pad*, and it gives us the round or apple shape to the cheek. These fat pads not only give our face it's plumpness and structure—functionally, they give padding and protection to important deeper structures like arteries and nerves. They make it easier for facial muscles to move against the soft, oily fat. For example, the *buccal fat pad*, which lies in front of your main chewing muscle (if you suck in your cheeks, it lies in that space), is thought to allow for easier movement and lubrication of the muscles during chewing.

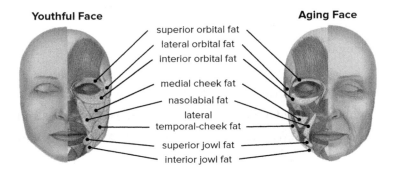

Deeper and beyond the loss of fat, shrinking of the bony skeleton has a huge impact on the way we look. As we age, the bones of the upper and lower jaws recede. The opening for the nose in the skeleton called the *pyriform aperture* widens. The bony orbits that house the eyes enlarge.

Young Female

Old Female

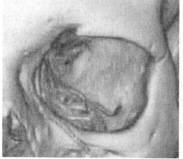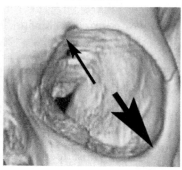

Robert B. Shaw, Evan B. Katzel, Peter F. Koltz, et al., "Aging of the Facial Skeleton: Aesthetic Implications and Rejuvenation Strategies," in *Plastic and Reconstructive Surgery* 127, no. 1 (January 2011): 374–83.

In the body, bony changes are perhaps more widely known, as many suffer from osteoporosis as they age, and broken long bones and hips with aging. People are well aware of the aging of the spine, as most older people have compression fractures and curving of the spine, resulting in a hunched-over gait.

In summary, aging is a gradual, insidious process, which involves aging of our cells on a microscopic (DNA) level and all of our organs on a macroscopic level. After we hit our "peak" in our early twenties, changes in our skin, fat, and bones begin to impact our outward appearance. Volume loss in the face and body begin first, then gravity takes hold in middle age. Aging seems to accelerate after the age of fifty, with our outward appearance reflecting our internal decline.

IS "NATURAL" BEST?

Now that you know a little more about the process of aging and its progression, let's talk more about whether this progression must be accepted as "natural." What exactly does aging "naturally" mean? We just discussed that aging is largely due to the aging of our cells, which happens with repeated division and accumulated mistakes in the DNA. This, of course, is a natural process, but we do all kinds of things to intervene, and so do our cells.

For example, cancers of all types are the result of cell division gone wrong. Cancer is essentially an error in a gene due to cell division, and the error leads to unchecked cell growth. Our bodies recognize this as an aberrancy and summon our immune system, most often successfully, to kill the abnormal cell or cells. However, when our immune system is unsuccessful and cancerous cells go unchecked, the microscopic (invisible/undetectable) disease becomes macroscopic (visible/detectable). Of course, while this process is natural, don't think twice about intervening with "unnatural" therapies like chemotherapy or radiation to alter the course of this natural event. Consider the focus of medicine on curing disease. Medicine, at its very core, is about altering the "natural" course of events. Therefore, by definition, medicine is unnatural if you define natural as "letting nature have its way."

Medicine inherently involves intervention, whether with procedures, therapies, or medications, to affect disease or alter the process of aging. The idea that one is more dangerous, scarier, or "wrong" because we're "altering a natural process" is downright ridiculous. Cosmetic surgery and aesthetic medicine are most subject to this objection, so many feel guilty about changing the way they look because they feel it is "unnatural" and defies the way aging should go. Aging gracefully is not synonymous with letting yourself go and letting nature take its course.

We take action medically when something malfunctions with our bodies, and we don't think twice about it. Aging is just a slower, more insidious malfunction of our cells, organs, and bodies on a massive scale, and aesthetic treatments and plastic surgery are just another way of intervening. They use the power of science and medicine to alleviate the malfunction of the skin, fat, muscle, and bone in our bodies that occurs with advancing age. If you feel better, younger, and more vital as a result, it's okay to use this form of medicine to fool Mother Nature.

THE MISCONCEPTIONS SURROUNDING "NATURAL"

Maybe it's not the thought of fooling with Mother Nature that has you worried, but the way that plastic surgery does it. Many are skeptical of medical science in general, and even more are fearful of plastic surgery. After all, what could be more unnatural or potentially toxic than cutting, stitching, putting toxins in your face, or having gel injected in your lips? It all sounds scary, unnatural, and, well, plastic. I completely understand where these misconceptions come from, but the reality is—and don't fall off the chair here—plastic surgery is as "natural" as any other form of medicine. It may be even more natural and safe than some of the other things you do to your body right now.

Do you take any natural supplements? I am sure for those who do, thinking about the "naturalness" of these compounds gives some reassurance about what they are putting in their bodies. But the definition of "natural" can be easily misconstrued, and the zeal that people have for living this lifestyle is sometimes confused and misplaced. I encounter this confusion on a daily basis. I may prescribe medication for a patient to prepare for surgery or to treat them for a particular condition.

To give an example, I prescribe a single antibiotic, which is similar to penicillin. Penicillin is a chemical produced by mold, which is pretty natural, although to get it into the proper form for consumption, it requires some processing.

Moreover, there are forty years of clinical studies and data proving the safety and efficacy of this potentially "poisonous" medicine. The potential side effects are well known and published on the packaging.

However, the hesitation, suspicion, and worry about taking a medicine is commonplace, particularly with patients who live a "natural" lifestyle. Frequently, these are also the patients who take supplements like ginko biloba, omega-3 fish oil, CoQ 10, St. John's wort, saw palmetto, and the list goes on and on.

Consider the process for natural supplements. Do they come straight out of the forest and onto your shelf? Don't they have to be altered and modified? Don't these "natural" products contain preservatives, additives, and God-knows-what-else so they could be put on shelves? What is considered to be a "natural" supplement is usually far from it.

Another striking difference between the medicines we use to alter the course of nature and natural supplements is clinical evidence that the substance you're ingesting is safe and effective. Drugs in this country go through a myriad number of hoops to scientifically prove their safety and efficacy. This is mostly regulated by the FDA, but is also done electively by companies to prove the worthiness of the drug to the larger medical community. With natural supplements or remedies, there is usually scant to absolutely no evidence that these natural supplements or remedies actually work.

Even scarier, if you are ingesting something that is "all natural" with little or no testing, how do you know it's actually safe? The body deals in the language of chemistry and biology, and it has no idea you have deemed this substance "natural." Plenty of substances in nature cause cancer, disease, and can even kill you (e.g., water hemlock, deadly nightshade, and tobacco).

How about those of you who take a boatload of natural supplements and remedies? We likely don't know how these various chemical substances interact with the body, because there is absolutely no information available on it. You're essentially rolling the dice when you take supplements. At least with medical drugs, the various interactions and potential complications of different combinations are well known and available for any pharmacist to reference.

In the world of plastic surgery, the interventions, injections, and drugs we use undergo rigorous testing and regulation. We know exactly what we are putting into people's bodies, and we know the potential side effects and complications. For example, perhaps one of the most feared and misunderstood drugs we use is Botox. Just the name, "Bo - **Tox**" inspires fear and suspicion. You may say, "Toxin in my body? No, thank you." However, Botox injections are the most common procedure done in all of cosmetic surgery. It's also probably one of the most studied, safest substances in all of medicine. It is a drug like any other that has a particular effect, and a safety profile that is well known.

Without boring you with too many details about Botox, it contains minute doses of a protein that the *Botulinim bacteria* produces. It blocks transmission between the nerves and muscles that are treated. The muscles relax, and wrinkles go away. The toxin is metabolized by the body in about three months, and the muscle returns to normal. Short-term side effects are extremely rare, and long-term ones are basically non-existent.

Perhaps you agree with my argument that plastic surgery treatments are based in medical science. But natural? "Come on, Doc!" Despite popular misconceptions, a lot of the things we do to make people look better are quite natural. There is a well-known philosophical principle in plastic surgery: "replace like with like." That means when something is missing (e.g., skin, muscle, fat, or bone), replace it with as close to the same tissue or substance as possible. I previously mentioned that a loss of facial fat and deflation of the facial fat pads occurs in facial aging. What do we do to replace this fat in facial plastic surgery? We add the exact same natural substance back into these fat pads— the patient's own fat—which is taken from another part of the body.

Similarly, you know the skin contains a tremendous amount of the substance hyaluronic acid, which giving the skin hydration and plumpness. You also know that the skin's ability to produce hyaluronic acid declines with age, leading to wrinkled, dry skin. So, what do we do to remedy this in facial plastic surgery? We inject fillers like Juvederm or Restylane, which contain natural hyaluronic acid, into the skin to fill in lines and wrinkles.

Let's examine another plastic surgery procedure: hair transplantation. In hair transplantation, we take a patient's own natural hair from areas where the hair is plentiful and transfer it to areas where hair was lost. While it may be a strange concept to think about, even plastic surgical procedures like facelifts, which involve cutting and stitching, work with natural principles. A well-done facelift follows the inherent dissection (separation) of planes of the face and repositions the fat, muscle, and skin back to their natural position before gravity took hold. Then, the body's healing mechanisms essentially hold everything in place. Many other plastic surgery procedures use the same principles.

The reality is, a lot of people experience guilt and worry about intervening in the aging process; they get this nagging feeling that maybe it isn't right to fool with Mother Nature. You may be one of them. Many objections you'll face when it comes to cosmetic surgery and non-surgical cosmetic procedures center around the idea that you should "age gracefully" (i.e., let yourself go). But now you know, on a biological level, the profound degradation and dysfunction of our skin, fat, and bone that comes with the passing of time. You know about the effects of gravity and the loss of volume in the process of aging. Based on the information you received in this chapter, you may have shifted your perspective of the aging process. It's not something that must be accepted as natural; it's a malfunction of our tissues that can be alleviated with plastic surgery and aesthetic medicine, just as other conditions can be alleviated by other forms of medical treatment.

I hope this chapter has helped you learn to question the idea of always equating "natural" with something that is **always** good for us, whether it's aging naturally or taking natural supplements. We explored the fear and skepticism you may be facing when considering plastic surgery because of popular misconceptions about what the treatments are. You learned that not only are the treatments based in proven medical science, but they can be a lot more natural in ways you never thought possible.

Do you have to let the aging process have its way in order to age gracefully? Some people have entirely different perspectives on what it means to "age gracefully," and different perspectives walk through my office doors. They have absolutely no fear about meddling with Mother Nature and intervening in any way possible to slow, reverse, or change the course of the aging and the effect it has on their appearance. For them, aging gracefully means the outside should look the way they feel on the inside. They take a proactive approach toward the aging problem and take advantage of the profound power of medical and surgical science to alter the course of aging.

It's not surprising that my patients also tend to be physically healthier than the average person of their age, as their proactive approach to aging leads to regular visits to the gym, taking care of their health, and more active lifestyles. Maybe looking and feeling as good as possible and doing all we can to maintain a young and vital appearance is a healthier approach to aging, and a more authentic way to "age gracefully."

8

Empowering Yourself to Look and Feel the Way You Want Safely and Effectively

So, maybe you're starting to view intervening in the aging process a little differently at this point. Now that you know about the degradation of the face and body on a biological level, you're starting to think: "What's wrong with steering Mother Nature in a better direction?"

Now you're also armed with a deeper understanding of the brain's interpretations of the aging process. You're past the anger of being judged for what you look like as you age, and understand that it's a function of our human brains to be visually judged by our appearance. You've accepted that the attractiveness advantage and ageism will impact your life whether you like it or not, and now you want to make the most of what you have. Maybe you're ready to take a more active role in your appearance and wellness. You've redefined "aging gracefully" from letting the aging process take over to maximizing what medical and surgical science has to offer. You may want to slow, reverse, or change the appearance of your aging face or body. So, where do you start? How do you do this safely and effectively? This chapter will cover some of the basics.

AVOIDING POTENTIAL PITFALLS

In the anti-aging and aesthetic industry, there are many potential pitfalls that patients need to avoid. The medical aesthetic industry is anticipated to reach $21 billion a year in 2024. This is an anticipated growth of 12 percent per year![23] The growth of the industry is fueled not only by the baby boomer population, but also by the surge of interest in these services by millennials and the younger generations. So, how much of this market is occupied by qualified medical doctors? Very little. Just like any other industry where demand is high, you will find a number of players who seek to take advantage of a trend. Lotions, potions, supplements, exercises, and procedures fill the aesthetic space that promise to make you "look years younger," with little to no scientific evidence that they actually work.

---

23   https://www.businesswire.com/news/home/20171023006050/en/
     Global-26.5-Billion-Medical-Aesthetics-Market-2024

In addition, numerous practitioners—doctors, dentists, physician's assistants, nurse practitioners, and nurses—with little to no training in plastic surgery have started providing aesthetic services in their spare time to supplement their incomes. In fact, the majority of medical spas, 60 percent, are now owned by people without board-certified, formal aesthetic training.[24] The pressure of waning insurance reimbursement for medical procedures has led these practitioners into the aesthetic space for the promise of cash-paying patients. A few weekend courses or a couple of seminars in neurotoxins, fillers, liposuction, or implants allow them to provide some of the same medical and even surgical services that I spent ten years in medical training to learn, and almost fifteen years in practice perfecting.

In the United States, medical tourism is a $20 billion-a-year industry and growing. The aesthetic market and demand for cosmetic surgery is growing at a rapid rate not only in this country, but also abroad, where there is an even higher concentration of untrained or unscrupulous providers. I get daily emails and "LinkedIn" requests from companies in China and Russia promising bargain basement prices on counterfeit Botox, fillers, sutures, and other products. Bargain basement prices entice some patients out of the country to have their cosmetic surgery, with medical tourism growing at an alarming rate. These overseas "clinics" offer

---

24 Alex R. Thiersch, JD, "The Rise of Non-Core Doctors, and What It Means," *Modern Aesthetics* (July/August 2018).

cosmetic surgery at a fraction of the price. Tragically, some of their patients pay the ultimate price, with the number of deaths, infections, and complications from medical tourism rising each year.

In the summer of 2019, three New Yorkers died in a three-week period after having procedures like liposuction, tummy tucks, and fat injections in the Dominican Republic. Pulmonary embolism, a clot in the arteries of the lungs, was the cause of at least one of those deaths. One major US medical center reported seeing seventy-eight patients over seven years who had serious complications from cosmetic plastic surgeries done abroad.[25] Using counterfeit materials under less than sterile conditions in the hands of an unqualified practitioner is a recipe for disaster. Let's cover some of the basics of how to get some work done in a way that is both safe and effective.

KNOW WHAT TO REASONABLY EXPECT

The old adage applies here: "If it sounds too good to be true, it probably is." Lotions, potions, and miracle creams sold on infomercials and by major department stores simply don't work. When I say they don't work, I mean they certainly won't make a major difference in your appearance. Yet the average American woman spends $313 a year on skincare

---

25   K. Ross, et al., "Plastic Surgery Complications from Medical Tourism Treated in a U.S. Academic Medical Center," *Plastic & Reconstructive Surgery* (2018).

products! A simple moisturizer can help the skin's appearance, but it won't provide the kind of life-changing, "wow" effect you are looking for.

You may have heard the term "cosmeceutical." These are lotions, potions, and creams that pose and position themselves as being able to treat conditions (e.g., wrinkles and brown spots). The Federal Food and Drug Agency says on its website, however: "The term 'cosmeceutical' has no meaning under the law. While the Federal Food, Drug, and Cosmetic Act (FD&C Act) does not recognize the term 'cosmeceutical,' the cosmetic industry uses this word to refer to cosmetic products that have medicinal or drug-like benefits. A product can be a drug, a cosmetic or both. The FD&C Act defines drugs as those products that cure, treat, mitigate, or prevent disease or that affect the structure or function of the human body. If a product makes such claims, it will be regulated as a drug. Cosmetics are intended to beautify, promote attractiveness, alter **appearance,** or cleanse; they are not approved by FDA for sale, nor are they intended to affect structure or function of the body."

The key word in the statement above is "appearance." That little piece of legal jargon is what allows companies to sell products as cosmetics and not as drugs. This means they can make all kinds of crazy claims without significant oversight or proof, as long as their claims are with regard to altering appearance. You may notice this in the small print on bottles or in the rapid, slick disclaimer in infomercials: "Improves the **appearance** of fine lines and wrinkles." Here, they cover their bases by telling you the product doesn't do what they just spent the entire commercial telling you it would do! Do you think the products you bought at Ulta, or the ones you bought for three installments of $19.95 from an infomercial, are going to do it? I think not. Save your money. It would be great if you could erase your bags, firm your neck, or tighten your jawline by applying a miracle cream at home, but you can't.

I recommend topical therapies to treat the skin all the time, but medical-grade products are different. What sets them apart from the myriad of lotions, potions, and creams? Two key differences: (1) they actually work, and (2) they are safe. Medical-grade products are sold directly to physicians. They are manufactured by companies with higher standards and back up their claims with scientific evidence in the form of clinical studies. These clinical studies are conducted in a controlled manner on volunteer patients to demonstrate the safety and second the efficacy of the product. So, you can be confident the medical-grade product will do what it actually says it does.

Medical-grade skincare products will improve wrinkles, fine lines, brown spots, and skin texture with prolonged and regular use, but not even they can cure your wrinkles.

SEEK THE RIGHT DOCTOR FOR YOUR INDIVIDUAL CONCERN

When you approach your anti-aging concerns, I recommend you first seek the counsel of a board-certified medical doctor who specializes in the area of your concern. I am, for example, a dual-board-certified facial plastic surgeon. My entire medical school, residency, and fellowship training (totaling ten years), as well as fifteen years in practice, have been focused on the head and neck. I am a face and neck specialist, and I perform more procedures in these areas, such as facelifts, eyelid lifts, and rhinoplasties, than your average cosmetic surgeon.

There are other specialties that focus on the surgical and non-surgical treatment of aging as well. The four main specialties form what we call the "core specialties," and the core specialists are facial plastic surgeons, plastic surgeons (who also treat the body), dermatologists, and oculoplastic surgeons (who specialize in the areas surrounding the eyes). While at times in history our professional organizations have been at odds, we agree that our background and educational training make our specialties uniquely qualified and suited to address each problem.

While you may find an occasional practitioner outside the core who has learned to provide excellent care through experience and trial and error, for the most part, my advice is to stick with a core provider. Doctors, dentists, nurse practitioners, physician's assistants, chiropractors, and any other provider outside the core likely obtained their training through a few weekend courses or company-sponsored trainings. They simply don't have the educational background to safely and effectively provide surgical or non-surgical cosmetic procedures. After all, cosmetic procedures are still *medical* procedures. And while complications and problems are relatively rare in good hands, they multiply in less than qualified hands. In addition, when complications or problems do arise, a practitioner without the proper experience and qualifications is less likely to recognize it and manage it appropriately.

DON'T BARGAIN SHOP FOR SURGICAL OR MEDICAL PROCEDURES

This brings us to another old adage: "You get what you pay for." While one might think it's common sense to value your face and body enough to elevate the purchase of medical and surgical procedures above that of a washing machine or flat-screen TV, there are people who greatly factor price into their decision-making equation. And there are bargain hunters out there by the bunches. They go to multiple lower-level providers to get prices and quotes, and hand over their faces and bodies to the lowest bidder.

I hope you are thinking: "That's ridiculous; I would never do that!" But in case you aren't, here's some more food for thought: providers of any kind who are cheap are cheap for a reason. They need to be. If they had the demand, above-board qualifications, an excellent reputation, and top-notch care commands, they would charge more. They simply don't provide the type of care that allows them to compete for patients who astutely value these factors over price. Instead, they entice the bargain hunters with their low, low prices.

Moreover, how do you think a provider might increase their profit while charging these low, low prices? In some cases, they cut corners. They may hire less-qualified people to support them, use lower-cost supplies, or maybe don't go to the trouble and expense of following the myriad number of costly required medical protocols, like sterilizing equipment properly.

So here, another old adage applies: *Caveat emptor* (buyer beware)! What are some red flags to look for when shopping for your cosmetic procedures? Groupons, plastic surgery chains, Botox parties in people's houses, numerous "flash sales," and spas with before-and-after pictures in your local *Penny Saver* are all to be avoided. Even the most qualified and reputable physicians do some promotions and discounts, but if the provider you are considering seems to be the "Walmart" of aesthetic procedures, it's probably best to steer clear. If you are going to someone's home or garage for the procedure, there might be a problem!

As we discussed earlier, going to another country for cosmetic surgery is not a good idea. Medical tourism is on the rise, and it is one of the fastest-growing global industries. In a report released by Visa and Oxford Economics in 2016, medical tourism was valued at $100 billion throughout the world, and it is expected to experience a 25 percent year-by-year growth by the year 2025. Unfortunately, the number of deaths and complications from people trying to get a deal outside the country is also on the rise. Over the years, a number of plastic surgery chains have come and gone, mostly due to the onslaught of lawsuits. They advertise a new "miracle medical procedure" (which is really surgery), offer "two for the price of one" deals on procedures, and massively advertise on TV. They even tout their "board-certified plastic surgeons." What kind of plastic surgeon would work for these corporations that offer rock-bottom prices? Remember, lower prices equal lower standards and a lower level of care.

Please don't misunderstand me—I am not arguing that you should be completely blind to price. After all, price is certainly a factor when you're making a purchase that can be quite expensive. My point is, once you have found a doctor or doctors who are, in fact, qualified to do your procedure, price should be the very last thing you factor into the equation. It is your face or your body, after all.

CHOOSING YOUR SURGEON: FACTORS TO CONSIDER

So, you have found a few board-certified, core physicians and you're considering having a procedure done. How do you choose, and what should factor into your equation? Here are a few good tips:

Inquire through word of mouth, or ask for referrals. Believe it or not, even in this day of at-your-fingertip digital information, word of mouth is still a pretty good way to find out information about your respective doctor, and it is the most common source of my referrals. Ask around, and usually someone you know will have gone to that particular physician, or someone will know of someone else who has. Tapping into a firsthand experience, particularly if it is with the same procedure you are interested in, can be invaluable. Granted, you may only find one or just a few opinions on this physician, so take it with a grain of salt if it is overly positive or negative, but it's a good place to start, at least.

In asking around, you will probably hear a community consensus on that particular physician. You might hear: "I've heard nothing but good things. He's an excellent doctor." Or, "I've seen him on TV and on the radio, but I've heard his practice is like a mill that churns out patients. I don't think he is very good or cares about his patients." Again, while the information is hearsay, it usually doesn't come from just one or two patients, but many, as community reputation is established throughout years of treating people.

And while I say again to take the information with a grain of salt, there is usually a grain of truth in a physician's community reputation.

Check online. Before you take the old-fashioned route of asking others about their experiences, you may want to head to the internet. Online reputation has become an even more important source of information for patients in search of their respective doctors. Google, Yelp, RealSelf, Healthgrades...there are a number of sources you'll want to look at and see how many stars and reviews there are for your physician. The more reviews, the more accurate the information. Your doctor should have an overwhelmingly positive online rating and near five stars. Note: near five stars, but not *exactly* five stars. If every review has five stars and there isn't a single negative word about the physician, I would be suspicious of the accuracy of the information.

Even the very best surgeons will have a few negative reviews. Some of these negative reviews might even be scathing with rambling, angry accounts of horrific outcomes, poor physician behavior, or staff transgressions. If there are a small number of negative reviews, no matter their content, again, take them with a grain of salt. Almost every physician encounters patients with unrealistic expectations or mental illness, or patients who were trying to manipulate the system for personal or financial gain. These patients are the most vocal, and usually the most angry and vindictive. Physicians are barred by privacy laws from responding with the details that may shed additional light on these cases, but the patient is allowed to provide any and all detail they would like, no matter how inaccurate. You may see "general" physician responses online for that reason.

INTERVIEWING YOUR PROSPECTIVE SURGEON

So, you've checked board certification, asked around your community, looked at your physician's online reputation, and decided to book an appointment. What additional information do you need, and what are important questions to ask before heading into the procedure room?

Ask about their skillset in your particular procedure. Experience or expertise in the particular procedure or procedures you are interested in is of utmost importance. Ask the surgeon how many of these procedures they perform in a typical week, month, or year. A week is the easiest timeframe, as the surgeon will know this at the top of their mind. Most surgeons will keep data on the number they perform in a year. If they are really on top of their game, they may know how many they perform against known national averages. That data is not easily accessible by the public, however. This is because most data on the number of surgeries performed for any procedure or specialty on a national level is kept by professional organizations and private companies. The data is usually given voluntarily by surgeons through surveys or polls, and so it may not be entirely accurate.

While you may not have the exact numbers for a particular procedure your surgeon performed to compare against a national database, you should know whether or not your surgeon performs the procedure you are interested in regularly and frequently. Their answer on the number of times they have done the procedure in a week, month, year, or overall should be provided with confidence and without hesitation.

Look at before-and-after images. Another good indication of the number of procedures a surgeon has performed is to look at their before-and-after pictures. Plastic surgery patients are usually hesitant to share their photographs and results with the public. Most patients prefer to keep the fact they have "had work done" completely confidential and will allow photography for their medical records only. Why do people prefer to hide images of their plastic surgery? Because of the core issue we discuss in this book: fear of being judged as vain, conceited, or superficial. Only about one in five patients will allow their before-and-after photos to be shown in the office, and even fewer allow it on social media and the internet. So, if you see ten high-quality "before-and-after" pictures, it may have taken fifty to one hundred patients to accumulate that many. But as a general rule, the more pictures you see, the more procedures a surgeon has performed. Obviously, quality matters just as much as quantity.

Here are a few key tips to follow when looking at before-and-after photos:

Look for consistency between the before photo and after photo. Lighting has a huge influence on the images you see before you. Is the lighting the same in both pictures? The appearance of facial aging in images is all about light and shadows. A picture that is washed out with soft lighting or flash will erase many facial flaws by eliminating shadows under the eyes, chin, and jawline. Conversely, a darker image will look more aged because it has more light and shadow contrasts. Make sure the before image isn't dark, and the after isn't flush with soft lighting. If the after image has more lighting than the before, it is not a reliable image on which to base your opinion.

Look at makeup. Is the patient not wearing makeup in the before image, but wearing makeup in the after? This is pretty obvious, but I mention it here to be complete. Makeup can make a huge difference in the of the appearance of before-and-after pictures; it can hide flaws and enhance pleasing features.

Look at the angles. What's the position of the head in the before-and-after images? The angle of the head tilt has a huge effect on the appearance of the face and neck. The more the chin is pointed down, the more gravity pulls on the face, and soft tissue gathers under the chin and in the neck. With the chin pointed down, eye bags look worse, smile lines deepen, jowls sag, and the neck will bunch. Lift the chin angle a few degrees, and voilà, the aging improves. Make sure the angle of the chin is consistent in the before-and-after photos.

Angles and positioning are equally important with regard to assessing body pictures. For example, if you're looking at liposuction of the abdomen, make sure the patient isn't exhaling in the before image and inhaling (sucking it in) in the after picture.

Lastly, when looking at before-and-after pictures, try to find someone whose problem and facial structure is similar to yours to assess real-life results. If you are considering rhinoplasty, look for a nose similar to yours to see what kind of results the surgeon was able to achieve on your type of nose. If you are having a facelift, look for someone who is roughly the same age, with some of the same problems. For example, if you have heavy jowls, deep smile lines, and a lot of neck skin, look at a before-and-after of someone ten years younger with mild jowls and a little neck laxity to see how successful your surgeon may be in your case. For body procedures, look for before images of people who have similar breasts or your body type.

Research the physician's malpractice cases. More than likely, the physician's community and online reputation will give you an accurate picture of their skill, competency, and safety, but you also want to examine the physician's malpractice history. If their history is excellent, they won't have an unusual number of lawsuits. But to be precise, you may want to check, and malpractice history is available through most state medical board websites or on the Administrators in Medicine (AIM) website, which is a non-profit organization that compiles physician malpractice and disciplinary information.

You may be surprised to find that it is quite normal for a physician of any experience to have some malpractice claims against them. We live in a tremendously litigious society, so physicians pay for malpractice insurance, which can cost in excess of $100,000 per year, per physician. I quote this number just to give you an idea of the scope of the problem. Lawsuits can be brought on quite frivolously with little cause, and some with the hope of financial gain. On average, a physician is sued once in every ten years of practice.[26] While accurate statistics aren't readily available, I suspect cosmetic surgeons are sued at a rate that is slightly higher than the average.

Here is how to interpret malpractice information:

---

26   G. Iacobucci, "GPs Can Expect to Be Sued Once Every 10 Years, MDU Warns," *BMJ* (2018): 362:k4016.

- **Look at the number and history of claims.** A few claims for a physician who has been in practice for twenty years is the rule, not the exception. But if a physician has ten or twenty claims for ten years of practice, this is definitely a red flag. For the claims they do have, you should also look at the claim history.
- **Look at the judgments.** Did they have a large judgment (money awarded the suing party) against them, or was it a small settlement? Larger judgments are an indication the judge or jury felt the case was an egregious case of malpractice. Small settlements are less serious, with physicians sometimes agreeing to settle just so they don't have to deal with the inconvenience of legal proceedings.
- **Check to see if the doctor was ever sanctioned.** It is also helpful to find out if the physician was ever sanctioned by an accrediting agency like a hospital or medical society.

WHAT DOES YOUR GUT SAY?

The last factor to consider, and this goes almost without saying, is how the physician and their office make you feel when you interact with them. The initial phone call, first visit to the office, and the initial meeting with the staff and physician will give you a sense of how they conduct themselves and the standards of care set from the top. What are the facilities like? How are you treated? Are important details given their due attention? After all, this is a place you are entrusting with your very person—your face or body. Your interactions should be professional with the highest standards, yet warm and caring. In my practice, we set the standard of treating patients like family (I am of Italian descent, after all), and we strive to offer a Ritz-Carlton-like experience. Since plastic surgery is elective surgery, I think it calls for these standards.

You can even ask the office if they have literature, or if a portion of their website describes their particular standards of care. If the office has no idea what you're talking about, perhaps they're not as focused on you, the patient, as they should be. Beyond your feelings about how you're treated at the office or by the staff, make note of your rapport with the treating physician. Physicians as a whole are not exactly known to be warm and fuzzy. As in any profession, we, of course, have many different personality types. However, physicians, and especially surgeons, are objective, factual, and have a tendency to use medical jargon. While a certain amount of this distancing or lack of connection serves a particular purpose in our profession (remember, objectification allows us to do our jobs), you want to discern between professional conduct and someone you just can't connect with.

Does the physician listen to you, or talk over or around you? Do they address and repeat your concerns back to you, or dismiss them? Do they seem sympathetic and caring, or cold and distant? Are they focused on delivering what you want, or selling you on procedures that you don't want? While some excellent surgeons with internationally known reputations are not selected for their bedside manner, choosing a physician without consideration for your rapport with them may leave you with a less-than-ideal cosmetic surgery experience. Don't underestimate your gut feelings when it comes to evaluating your choice of an office or surgeon. You're going through a very personal journey and perhaps the formation of a long-term relationship.

In this chapter, we covered some of the pitfalls to avoid as well as important factors to consider now that you've decided to pursue a procedure or treatment to look and feel younger. Lotions, potions, infomercials, plastic surgery chains, unqualified practitioners, discount plastic surgeons, and medical tourism are several things to be wary of, and it's generally a good idea to avoid them completely. Seeking out a board-certified core physician (facial plastic surgeon, plastic surgeon, dermatologist, or oculoplastic surgeon), checking community and online reputation, gauging the number of procedures performed, looking at before/after images critically, and screening malpractice history are all great steps to ensure that you've performed your due diligence. Finally, don't underestimate your gut feeling on how the physician and office make you feel. A good relationship is an important component of the experience with your non-surgical or surgical cosmetic procedure.

9

Real Patient Stories

In this chapter, I would like to share some excerpts of stories from my actual patients. You will see some of the central themes and ideas presented in this book played out in real life. Some patients struggled with their initial guilt; worried about vanity, lack of support, and plastic surgery shaming; and experienced feeling bad about wanting to look good firsthand. You will see how for some their physical flaws caused intense emotional and psychological limitation and pain. Themes you have learned about in this book, like the visual/social nature of human interaction, self-image formation, ageism, and the attractiveness advantage, are present in many of the stories these patients shared about their plastic surgery experiences. Ultimately, in sharing their intimate stories of physical and emotional transformation, these generous souls will demonstrate how physical appearance can have a great impact on the way others see us, and the way we see ourselves.

Here is an excerpt from one patient story. "After the sudden loss of my husband, my physical appearance changed. I work in the beauty industry as a hairstylist and makeup artist, and I took about eight months off. This wasn't because of how I looked, but because I didn't want to be social or talk about him with clients. After seeing pictures of myself with my granddaughters, I realized I was wearing the pain on my face and in my eyes. This change in appearance along with significant weight loss made me look like a melted candle. I didn't want to be constantly reminded of my pain every time I looked in a mirror. I just wanted it to go away."

From another patient: "The two years prior to my surgery were terrible. I lost my dear mother and my husband. I was caregiver to both. I couldn't care for my husband during the last month of his life because I had been diagnosed with cancer and was recovering from a mastectomy. Talk about poor timing! After a period of grief, physical recovery, and reconstruction, I found myself with poor body image and low self-esteem. I literally needed a lift! My sister had just undergone facial surgery and was very pleased with the results. I chose to have some as well. I definitely felt guilt. Why should I be so vain? I should just be happy to be a two-time cancer survivor!"

This patient also said: "I don't like to feel judged, and I know a lot of people are against cosmetic surgery, but aging makes me sad. I feel powerless. I decided just as I color my hair and do my nails, it's my right to have plastic surgery and feel more like myself again. I don't care about the rest. Deep inside, I know everyone enjoys looking at a beautiful face… it's like looking at art! The days of recovery after surgery were scary. I thought, "What if I look too different? What if I don't heal well? What if I don't look better at all?" I prayed things would turn out the way I expected, and they did! I feel much better. I can't wait to do another surgery when I have the time and money. I don't have to think about how old my eyes look anymore, and fewer negative thoughts means more positive thoughts. That is a win!"

From a third patient: "To an extent, yes [I felt guilt]. I told myself at a young age to love myself exactly as I was, but as I got older, I realized I wasn't putting forward the best version of myself. My nose was causing me to hide from things I loved." After the surgery: "It feels like I am looking at a new person in the mirror. My self-confidence is greater than it's ever been, and now I do things I never would have done with my 'old nose.' Taking photos doesn't scare me or make me feel insecure. I can touch the bridge of my nose without pain, and the drooping of the tip is gone, so you can actually see me smile. I'm a completely new woman! The surgery inspired me to better myself in all aspects of my life. Loving how I look has taught me to generally love myself more. I remember when the cast came off, and I went home. It was my twenty-first birthday! My mom looked at me, smiled the biggest smile I've ever seen, and said: 'I've never been able to see that part of your face before.' This was because of the drooping of the tip of my nose."

A fourth patient story: "I was in my mid-sixties and I didn't recognize the old lady in the mirror. The thought of a facelift was the last thing I wanted, so I explored other options that did not require general anesthesia. I had no idea who to ask for ideas and guidance, so I took to the internet. One name kept popping up at the top of every search: Dr. James Marotta. I was unable to find a negative comment about him, so I took a deep breath and made an appointment for a consultation. I asked about every alternative to a facelift, but Dr. Marotta was honest and said the only thing that would make me happy was a facelift. I had been dead set against doing that, but I walked out with a surgical appointment.

Dr. Marotta made me feel confident and dispelled any fears I had. The decision to have a facelift is one of the best I have ever made for myself. I was constantly depressed about my looks and avoided mirrors at all costs. There was probably a two-year period where I hardly looked at myself. My mental well-being took precedence over any other issues.

People knew I had the procedure, and they were astonished at how well it turned out. To this day, if I see people I haven't seen in years, they say how wonderful and young I look. I look very natural and not "plastic," and no one knows I had any work done. Since my surgery, I am constantly surprised when I catch a glimpse of myself in the mirror and I like what I see. My entire outlook on life has gotten so much better. I have lost a bit of weight and feel better than I have in years. I had not seen my sister in fourteen years as she lives in Florida, and neither one of us was willing to travel. About six months after my surgery, my niece was getting married and I couldn't miss the wedding. I bit the bullet and traveled to Florida. My sister came to the hotel where I was staying, and I waited for her at the elevator. When the doors opened, she saw me and exclaimed: 'I can't believe it, you look exactly the same as you did the last time I saw you!' P.S. I never told her. LOL."

There are so many more patient stories I could share. Thank you from the bottom of my heart to the patients who volunteered their stories to help people who are perhaps struggling with their decision to have plastic surgery.

Conclusion

Remember Valerie? We started this book with her story. She was seeking cosmetic surgery, but she was racked with the guilt, fear, and trepidation that can accompany this journey. Resistance from family, friends, and the world had her "feeling bad about trying to look good." She overcame the personal and public shaming, and transformed her appearance and her life.

In the second chapter, we explored some of the reasons why people face such public and private resistance when it comes to plastic surgery. We talked about the negative stigma of plastic surgery in America, rooted in our puritanical sensibilities, and bolstered by the negative attention on TV and the internet. We learned, however, that the media's fascination with the grotesque and macabre is really more of a plastic surgery fantasy than reality. The rest of the world and most cultures have an entirely different view of plastic surgery and physical transformation; it's more positive and life-affirming.

In the third chapter, we talked about common fears surrounding plastic surgery procedures: fear of complications, fear of the results not matching expectations, fear of looking like a celebrity disaster, and fear of being "botched" or becoming a plastic surgery addict. We learned that plastic surgery complications and problems are rare, and the exception rather than the rule. Bad outcomes can be influenced much more by patient choices to have certain procedures or multiple procedures, rather than dictated by a single surgery or a single surgeon's slip of the knife.

Following that discussion, we delved into how to determine if you or a loved one are taking it too far with plastic surgery. I shared with you the thought process and struggle that I have as a physician charged to "do no harm," or more like, "only do perfect," in choosing patients appropriately. Identifying someone who is unrealistic or taking it too far with plastic surgery is a lot more difficult than it seems at face value, because human beings are complex. Despite this complexity, we discussed the importance of identifying someone with true mental illness or Body Dysmorphic Disorder (BDD), and looked at the behavior they exhibit along with some of the warning signs. These patients should not have cosmetic surgery.

Outside of patients with a clear diagnosis of BDD, obsessive behaviors regarding a particular body part or feature are clearly on the rise. The lines whether to operate or not operate, inject or not inject, are becoming even more blurred. The digital age, the rise of social media, and the selfie have brought a new focus on looking perfect, filtered, and flawless. The attractiveness advantage is amplified and multiplied by the instantaneous feedback through likes and views on social media, with the younger generations leading the charge to prevent, enhance, and perfect through cosmetic surgery and non-surgical procedures.

I shared with you the personal "line" that I do not cross when patients ask me to create a look I don't feel is natural or attractive. Yet even that line gets blurred when I'm asked to cover or correct years of previous cosmetic surgery or non-surgical intervention that cannot necessarily be reversed. The bottom line is that cosmetic surgery "nightmares" are the exception rather than the rule. They won't happen to you if you do your research, find a qualified surgeon, and make a conscious choice toward improvement and not perfection, natural and not ubernatural.

In chapter 4, we started to uncover why choosing to change one's appearance is not such a "vanity purchase" (pun intended) after all. We delved into the biological and sociological underpinnings of why we do (and should) care greatly about the way we look. There is a connection between looking good and feeling good that we cannot so easily divide. We also explored the human brain and how we form opinions of others based on how they look. The human brain evolved to make snap judgments about facial appearance to keep us safe from threat and disease. In the brain, there is a tremendous amount of space and power dedicated to the processing of human faces.

We looked at self-image and how it is formed at a very early age by what our closest family members tell us about our appearance. Our self-image is also greatly influenced by how we appear to others (i.e., our defining physical characteristics). Physical judgment is part of every social interaction from cradle to grave. In this light, it makes absolutely no sense to deny that your physical appearance is important to you, or to others around you. It makes no sense to have any guilt or shame when considering cosmetic surgery or non-surgical procedures. Plastic surgery patients astutely recognize that you cannot separate how you look from how you feel. In this light, cosmetic surgery and other interventions are not only pragmatic, but are a way of displaying and reflecting the health, vitality, and beauty that you feel on the inside to the outside world.

In chapter 5, we tried to rein in the anger and objections that some potentially still have regarding plastic surgery. They believe undergoing a procedure is "giving in to objectification" because you let others treat you as an object to be looked at and evaluated. We explored the concept of objectification and what it truly means to treat another human being as an object. We found out, however, that a much larger amount of human communication is visual and subliminal than we realize, and caring about your appearance is not giving in to objectification. It is recognizing and capitalizing on the fundamental fact that human beings communicate visually.

We then discussed whether or not the drive to have plastic surgery was driven in part by sexism, given that 90 percent of cosmetic surgery patients are women. While certainly, a double standard does exist when it comes to judging women on their appearance, the reasons women choose to have plastic surgery are based in biology. Women have a higher visual/social sense, and they are more in tune to the visual/ social feedback they receive about the way they look, not only from men, but also from other women. Because women value social feedback more, they are happier when they look their best.

Yet another biological reason women may be more pre- disposed toward cosmetic enhancement has to do with differences in the aging faces of women versus men. Despite a clear sexist double standard, men do tend to be a bit more biologically insulated from the effects of aging. This is due to the thickness of their skin and the size of their facial skel- eton. The bottom line is, seeking cosmetic enhancement does not need to be viewed as giving in to objectification or a sexist double standard; rather, it is recognizing biological/

social realities and empowering oneself to maximize their appearance to their social advantage.

We also examined the blurred lines between basic grooming, medical necessity, and "radical plastic surgery." While no one gets shamed for performing basic grooming tasks, people frequently get shamed when they enter into cosmetic alteration and enhancement. People who have plastic surgery are not vain, conceited, self-centered, or insecure—they have a healthier, more pragmatic attitude about their appearance. Plastic surgery patients take charge of their appearance, and this can be viewed as mentally and physically healthy, just like taking care of yourself through exercise, diet, healthy habits, or meditation.

In chapter 6, we went even further with this point. We discussed that optimizing your appearance is not only mentally and physically healthy, but may offer you a distinct advantage in life and in your social interactions. There is an "attractiveness advantage" that is a pervasive and well-established principle of human social interaction. Physical traits can and are interpreted heuristically (in the blink of an eye) by the brain, and ascribed either positive or negative meaning based on their attractiveness.

We looked at certain facial features and their social interpretations (e.g., weak chin equals mousy, strong chin equals assertive), what is considered to be the aesthetic ideal, and what is considered less than ideal for various facial features. The attractiveness advantage is hardwired into the brain, as we saw with the example of babies preferring to gaze at attractive faces, because they interpret those faces as healthier and more capable of providing for their needs. The attractiveness advantage is a pervasive fact of adult life, as we saw with the example of height conveying an electability advantage for both American presidents and CEOs of companies.

The attractiveness advantage is also an obvious factor when it comes to choosing a mate. Attractiveness is interpreted as being biologically healthy and having worthy genes to pass on to offspring. The attractiveness advantage can factor into the decisions made about us and the likelihood of our success in almost every sphere of life. We see it in Hollywood, in the political stage, in the media, and in business. The harsh reality is that the attractiveness advantage declines with advancing age, and we talked about the prevalence of ageism both in the workplace and in our interpersonal lives.

With regard to age, we elucidated the heuristic interpretations the brain gives to certain aging facial features (e.g., eye bags equals tired). Given the importance of physical appearance and vitality to our social interactions and our possibility of success, you should make no apologies, and feel no guilt or twinge of vanity, over maximizing the attractiveness advantage through any means possible at any stage in your life. The bottom line is, it's smart to care about the way you look.

We then explored the false choice between "aging gracefully" and "aging naturally." For some, aging gracefully means avoiding any kind of intervention, whether a minimally invasive procedure or cosmetic surgery, and letting "nature have its way." Others in an effort to "age naturally" turn toward "natural" or homeopathic cures, which can have little or no known medical benefit, and can even possibly be harmful.

An alternative view is to deny that aging is natural at all, and we dove deep into the process of aging. You learned about aging from a cellular level, to the level of the tissues (i.e., skin, fat, bones, muscles), to the macroscopic level of age-related changes in the structures of the face and body. We learned that these changes in the cells and tissues reflect degradation and dysfunction, which is a hallmark of pathology or disease. The degradation and dysfunction of cells and tissues that occurs as a result of aging is what leads to a change in our outward appearance. In any other form of medicine, we intervene, manipulate, and alter what has gone awry with optimal physiologic function. Aesthetic medicine and plastic surgery are no different than any other form of medicine. They seek to alter the "natural" course of events for a healthier, more optimal function and appearance.

Many people take a different perspective and select the

alternative way to "age gracefully." They take advantage of all that medical science, aesthetic medicine, and plastic surgery have to offer to modify the aging process. It's not surprising these patients also tend to be healthier physically than the average person, and perhaps they are the true bearers of the torch to age gracefully.

Chapter 7 was written for those who had been impacted by the information they gained earlier in this book about the aging process, the visual/social nature of the human brain, the attractiveness advantage, and ageism. A roadmap was presented for those who were perhaps ready to move beyond their initial objections, trepidation, and even anger at the prospect of cosmetic surgery or a non-surgical procedure. They are ready to take an active role in their appearance and wellness.

We answered many important questions about pursuing plastic surgery in this chapter. What are the first steps to approach cosmetic surgery or a non-surgical procedure? How do you do it safely and effectively? What are some of the pitfalls to avoid? We also looked at the aesthetic industry in the United States as a booming business with a number of players offering cosmetic medical services without the proper training and qualifications. We discussed the dangers of counterfeit products from China and Russia, and why it is best to avoid traveling to another country for cosmetic surgery.

We discussed the cosmeceutical industry and how the claims many products make are based on little or no science. Remember, if it is cheap, bargain basement, found in a penny saver, or "too good to be true" for cosmetic surgery, run, don't walk, in the other direction. A safer approach is to seek a board-certified surgeon or medical doctor who specializes in your area of concern from one of the four "core" specialties. Cheaper equals less expertise, less training, less overhead, and a higher likelihood of a poor result or, even worse, a complication. *Caveat emptor* (buyer beware)!

We also talked about what to do when you find a qualified surgeon. We discussed how to properly vet your practitioner: find out their reputation through word of mouth and online reviews. Find out their level of experience or expertise for the procedure you are considering, look at before-and-after photos, examine their malpractice history, and go with your gut feeling in your dealings with the physician and the office. These are all factors that must be considered.

Finally, I shared actual stories of patients who wrestled with their decision to pursue cosmetic surgery. They were gracious and kind enough to share their very intimate and personal thoughts on how their appearance deeply affected their self-image and happiness. You learned of the positive changes surgery or cosmetic procedures brought not only to their appearance but to their entire outlook on life.

I hope you enjoyed this book and that it helped, in some small way, to alleviate any stress, guilt, or angst you have (or have had) in pursuing cosmetic surgery or non-surgical procedures. You should not have to feel bad about wanting to look good. I hope this book convinced you that improving yourself by using the best medical science has to offer is pragmatic, healthy, empowering, and frankly a smarter approach to aging than letting Mother Nature have her way. Ignore the shamers and naysayers, and feel free to share the information in this book with them.

If you struggled with your decision to move forward with your cosmetic surgery or non-surgical procedure, my staff and I would love to hear your story. Please share your Transformational Experience™ with us at MarottaMD.com, and continue the conversation in our private Facebook group. We and other patients would love to hear how you overcame your deepest fears or harshest critics to transform your life through your cosmetic surgery or non-surgical procedure(s). Share your story, your before-and-after photos, or even videos if you feel comfortable. If you have questions, ask away. We're all here to help. This is a shame/judgment-free, positive forum where you will find the support and help you need.

Acknowledgments

I would like to thank Scribe Guided Author and Lioncrest Publishing, Tucker Max, Hal Clifford, Ellie Cole, and Nicole Jobe for their guidance and help in writing my first book. I would like to thank the members of my Marotta Plastic Surgery Specialists team for their work and support on the book, including Sharon Marotta, Sarah Corallo, Alisa Vinasco, Katie Lave, and Niki Castagna. Thank you, Sharon, for your work in the read-aloud edit, and for your perspective and suggestions that made the book better. A special thanks to my executive assistant, Sarah, who worked many hard hours researching articles, references, and pictures, and who endured the final stages of the read-aloud edit. Alisa, thank you for helping me make the book have a larger impact. To my parents and sister, Lucille, Samuel Marotta, and Michelle Marotta, thank you for your love and support throughout my life, for making me the man I am, and for showing me the value of hard work. Thank you to my mother-in-law, Joan Costa Arlen, for believing in me, loving me, and helping me get the practice off the ground. To my children, Noah and Gillian Marotta, words can never express the extent of Daddy's love for you, the depth of my pride, or my belief in both of you. Find what you love, dream big, work hard, and all things are possible.

Appendix: The Most Important Points to Remind Yourself of When Doubts Occur

The main purpose of this book is to provide support for those who are struggling with decisions surrounding plastic surgery. I wrote this book for patients who are conflicted and feel the guilt, worry, or shame that can be associated with pursuing plastic surgery or non-surgical enhancement. There are many other issues you may be wrestling with and arguments you may be facing within yourself or from others. To that end, here is a recap of points you can revisit when you face those arguments, or you feel doubtful or conflicted.

Chapter 1: Valerie's Story

- In the months since her surgery, Valerie feels like a different person.
- She can't believe she walked around like that for so long. She can't believe she felt so badly about herself for so many years.
- Does that sound like you? Could it potentially be your story?

Chapter 2: The Guilt and Shame over Plastic Surgery in America: For the Vapid, Vain, and Deformed

- "Plastic" in plastic surgery has nothing to do with the material, a fake appearance, or being man-made. "Plastic" comes from the Greek word *plastikos*, meaning "to mold or change."
- In many cultures throughout the world, plastic surgery is celebrated and even venerated as life-affirming and empowering, without any of the negative bias or associations it has in America.
- The history of cosmetic enhancement dates back to Ancient Egypt—at least in recorded history—and is probably as old as time. Wanting to improve one's appearance and taking action to do so seemed to be important to human beings throughout history. Cosmetic surgery is embraced and celebrated by many cultures in the world today, without any of the social condemnation or negative repercussions you see in America.

Chapter 3: Fear: Why Does Plastic Surgery Go Wrong or Too Far?

- Serious complications or problems *should be* exceedingly rare. However, I suggest you ask your prospective cosmetic surgeon or practitioner about any serious complications in their practice.
- Because drama sells, the worst-case scenarios are featured most prominently on reality TV, the internet, and tabloids.
- Plastic surgery "disasters" constitute an extremely small percentage of plastic surgery patients and plastic surgery cases. They capture our attention because we can't help but notice them.
- There are a huge number of plastic surgery patients living among you. You see them on the streets, in the stores, and on your movie screens, TV screens, and computers. They have results that are beautiful, natural, and undetectable. You don't notice them because the results are *beautiful, natural, and undetectable*.
- The plastic surgery nightmares you see in the media, on the internet, and in Hollywood are frequently the result of a vicious cycle where the patient wants something more or something different, and has multiple procedures. Michael Jackson's nose was not the result of one or two surgeries with a few surgeons, but the result of multiple surgeries with multiple surgeons over a period of years.
- Patients with Body Dysmorphic Disorder (BDD) should not have cosmetic surgery. However, these patients only

comprise a small percentage of patients (from 2 to 10 percent).

Chapter 4: The Connection between Looking and Feeling Good
- Your physical and emotional aspects both deserve love and attention. The two are interconnected. When we feel that we look our best, it translates internally to augment our feelings of confidence and vitality. Together, they work to support each other to form the picture of who we perceive ourselves to be.
- Recall how you felt when you had a monster zit as a teenager. Now compare that with how you felt after it was gone. Plastic surgery can accomplish the same type of transformative results.
- When we see someone with anything "wrong" with their face (e.g., a deformity, a burn, big eye bags, sunken cheeks, even really bad wrinkles), the truth is we cannot help but stare a bit as we try to interpret the situation. We get a strange sense we should avoid the interaction. When we see someone with an attractive or, as we learned, strikingly average face, we might also stare, but usually with the opposite vibe. We are attracted to, and sympathetic toward, the beautiful face. This reaction is hardwired in our human brains.

Chapter 5: Changing Your Appearance through Plastic Surgery Is Not Giving In to Objectification, Sexism, or Extremism

- Caring about how you look is not giving in to objectification or inviting people to consider you only on the basis of your appearance. It is capitalizing on the fundamental fact that human beings communicate visually. Instead of feeling like you are giving in or selling out by changing the way you look to make yourself or others happy, why not see it as empowering yourself to communicate your inner beauty, inner strength, and inner vitality to the world in the way that most human beings will first and foremost receive that information?

- The drive for women to appear beautiful to the world is rooted in biology and evolution. Women have a more powerful visual/social sense.

- Men, on average, show signs of facial aging more slowly than women.

- Women feel it is important to look good not only to please men, but to please each other, and most importantly, to please themselves. Ironically, in this sense, embracing the idea of maximizing appearance through non-surgical treatments or plastic surgery may be viewed as more female or even, dare I say, "feminist."

- People have plastic surgery for some of the very same reasons we wash our hair, cut our nails, and generally take care of the way we present ourselves. Although plastic surgery is a bit more involved than combing our hair, no one takes issue with or judges someone for combing their hair. No one gets shamed because they regularly take showers, but the plastic surgery patient must frequently hide, lie, conceal, and cover for fear of social retribution from friends or family.

- Most people who have plastic surgery are grounded, healthy people who have something they simply want to improve about their appearance.

Chapter 6: The Attractiveness Advantage: Why It's Smart to Care about How You Look

- The attractiveness advantage is not learned, but appears to be hardwired into our brains. Even babies judge faces according to their beauty and show a clear, discernible preference for gazing at attractive faces. They are being biologically practical.

- Consider how witches' noses are portrayed versus how the nose of a princess is drawn. The brain ascribes meaning to bodily features based on the shape, size, and configuration of those features.

- The attractiveness advantage plays a part in almost every sphere of human interaction. Physical attractiveness is one of the most important factors for men and women in courtship and mating.

- Attractiveness also plays a part in our career success, with Hollywood being the most obvious example. Even outside of TV and movies, multiple studies have shown that for every inch of height above the average, that person earns an additional 1.8 percent in annual wages.

- "Negative physical traits diminish earning power. Shorter-than-average men receive 4 percent less in salary than those with average height, and obese women suffer a 5 percent loss in wages. General unattractiveness brings a wage loss in the range of 7 to 9 percent."
- Studies indicate that the visible signs of aging reflect physiologic or biological age and are independent of chronological age. Therefore, looking old is a clear and accurate sign (and an accurate sign to others) that you are, in fact, less healthy, less vital, and perhaps less capable.
- If you are seeking to improve your appearance at any age, whether through diet, exercise, non-surgical intervention, or plastic surgery, you are making the smarter play. There is nothing wrong with wanting your outward appearance to reflect your inner health, vitality, and zest for life. You are maximizing your attractiveness advantage, which can have profound effects in every aspect of your life.

Chapter 7: The Guilt over Defying Nature: Why Aging "Gracefully" Doesn't Always Mean "Naturally"

- Should we let "nature have its way"? Is plastic surgery "unnatural"? Cancer is a "natural" process, but we don't think twice about intervening with "unnatural" therapies like chemotherapy or radiation to alter the course of this natural event. In fact, consider the entirety of medicine and its focus on curing disease. Medicine, at its very core, is about altering the "natural" course of events. Therefore, by definition, medicine is unnatural if you define natural as "letting nature have its way."

- Botox injections are the most common procedure done in all of cosmetic surgery. It is probably one of the most studied and one of the safest procedures to have in all of medicine. It's a drug like any other that has an effect and safety profile that is well known.

Chapter 8: Empowering Yourself to Look and Feel the Way You Want Safely and Effectively

- Know what to reasonably expect: if it sounds too good to be true, it probably is. Be wary of "miracle creams," unreasonable promises, cheap plastic surgery, and the like.
- Conduct diligent research for any procedure or physician you are considering.

I'd like to remind you that you should not have to feel bad about wanting to look good. I hope this book has convinced you that seeking to improve yourself using the best that medical science has to offer is pragmatic, healthy, empowering, and frankly a smarter approach to aging than letting

Mother Nature have her way. Ignore the shamers and nay-sayers and feel free to share the information in this book with them.

About the Author

DR. JAMES C. MAROTTA is a dual-board-certified facial plastic surgeon on Long Island, New York, with degrees from some of the world's finest institutions, including Columbia and Yale Universities. Dr. Marotta is a fellow of the American Academy of Facial Plastic and Reconstructive Surgery (AAFPRS), and since 2013, he has consistently been named the Best Cosmetic Surgeon on Long Island. Dr. Marotta has appeared in a variety of TV and print media, including *Harper's Bazaar, Huffington Post,* and Fox 5 NY.

While he is deeply dedicated to his work, family remains the center of Dr. Marotta's life. He enjoys spending time with his wife and two children, traveling, playing sports, and cooking.